Dear friend, I pray that you may enjoy good health and that all may go well with you, even as your soul is getting along well.

(3 John 2, NIV)

Contents

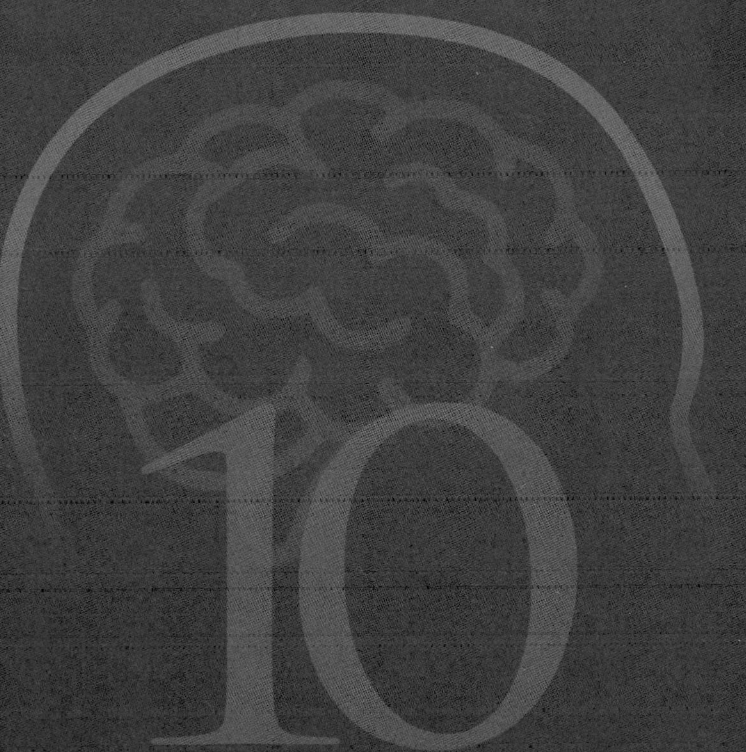

10 HABITS *of* WELLNESS

FOR A HAPPIER AND HEALTHIER LIFE WITH LESS ILLNESS AND DISEASE

MICHAEL ELLISON

10 Habits of Wellness
– For a Happier and Healthier Life with Less Illness and Disease

Published by TriVita Press

ISBN: 978-1-943157-78-5

Printed in the United States of America

To order go to:
www.TriVita.com

Why Are You Here?

When you walk into our TriVita clinic of Integrative Medicine, you are greeted by a question beautifully presented on a wall of stones. It simply reads:

Why are you here?

Some patients are offended because getting past their pain or illness seems to be the obvious answer. They have never thought beyond the point of their ailment, but the patients who search deeper for an answer to the question soon realize how the power of purpose and meaning actually helps with their healing and well-being. They connect the care of whole person and meaning of life with their health and well-being, and as a direct result, they typically have a far greater healing experience.

Many physicians, such as Dr. Wayne Jonas, author of the book *How Healing Works*, understand the significant difference between *curing* and *healing*. They recognize that the meaning and purpose of life is intrinsically connected to the healing process, and that includes all the physical, emotional, and spiritual elements of life as well. When people focus on their purpose and their overall wellness, rather than just the cure for their illness or disease, there is almost always a better outcome!

In truth, the absence of disease does not necessarily mean you have the optimal life of wellness and purpose that God planned for you. God desires for you to have abundant life! Like it says in 3 John 2, *"Dear friend, I pray that you may enjoy good health and that all may go well with you, even as your soul is getting along well"* (NIV).

God has designed you for wellness and purpose. David in the Psalms wrote, *"I praise you because I am fearfully and wonderfully made; your works are wonderful, I know that full well"* (Psalm 139:14).

You might not feel wonderful right now, and that's okay. Or you might feel pretty good but would much rather feel wonderful! Whatever your starting point, you will benefit from learning the habits of wellness!

Habit behavior (both good and bad) has been studied at most major universities over the past decades. Massachusetts Institute of Technology (MIT), for example, has a department committed to studying the habit loop behavior. Numerous books have come from these studies, such as the *New York Times* best seller *The Power of Habit*, which provides scientific validation of the power of habit behavior.

Habits are an integral part of health and wellness by the simple fact that we all do what we want to do. When our habits are good and they benefit our bodies, then we are on our way! But if our habits are bad, our bodies pay a price. What we need to do is replace the bad habits with good ones.

Habit formation is a powerful and vital part of not only our wellness but of our enjoyment of life as well. Life is easier when we don't have to think so hard, spending energy and mental focus trying to do what we know we should be doing.

When good behavior becomes habitual, we get good rewards with very little work! The habit creation process is simplified when we use reminders, routines, and rewards. When you put those three Rs to work for you, the good choices and good habits are so much easier to make. And you get what you want!

My intention is to help you do just that, and that entails creating wellness habits that contribute to a happier and healthier life with less illness and disease.

I have learned that wellness is not a single place or destination but a life journey. On that journey, you address questions such as:

- Who am I?
- Why do I matter?
- How can I support the wonderful person that God created me to be?

Having this mindset, establishing habits of wellness is a process. It will take some time and effort to work through and develop more insight on your journey, to clarify your answers to each of these questions.

No matter what condition of health or wellness you may be in, you can have even greater wellness. That is always the case. God designed your amazing body to work, to heal itself, and to keep you well.

Wellness is both a desired goal as well as a reward. To me, and as I use wellness throughout the book, wellness means:

> To have the vitality and energy to do the things you love and purpose to do, to have daily positive emotions of love, forgiveness,

gratitude, and acceptance, and to feel connected to God and His purpose for your life.

Our wellness is a state of being that is typically in fluctuation due to the experiences life offers us. The 10 habits of wellness described here will help guide us in our priorities in responding to life situations.

I invite you to go on your wellness journey with a mindset to discover and embrace the nutrients and nurturing essentials of wellness. You will be amazed at the results you will receive.

You have great purpose, purpose that goes beyond yourself and gives meaning to you and to others. The wellness that your body was created to enjoy is what enables you to fully live out your purpose.

The reason why you are here is your own lifelong mission ... and the purpose of the 10 habits of wellness is to help you do just that!

Foreword

Our country is in trouble! So many people are suffering from lifestyle-related chronic diseases. Processed foods, sedentary lifestyles, and relational and cultural issues are robbing us of our wellness. And people are falsely reassured by the medical establishment that they will be cured with a pill, procedure, or surgery!

With that as their go-to plan, millions of Americans charge into middle age denying and ignoring their physical and emotional needs. This lack of awareness leads to premature disability and disease.

When people wake up to the fact that there is no pill, procedure, or surgery that will meet their needs, most resign themselves to living out their lives in pain, limited in what they can do with thwarted hopes and dreams.

This doesn't have to happen, and Michael Ellison is committed to making sure it doesn't … one life at a time. Having lived out this common delusion, he awoke barely able to function and without a solution from modern medicine. Armed with his deep faith, loving wife, family, and a passion to live a full life, he set out to discover how to regain his vitality and to heal his body.

Contained in this book are the discoveries he has successfully shared with hundreds of thousands of Americans on how to reclaim their lives. Very early in the process, and before most medical experts had any appreciation for it, he discovered that focusing on healing the physical body was not enough – the body, mind, and spirit must all be recruited for true healing. These three life energies (tri-vitas) working together provide the foundation of transformation and whole health.

As a medical doctor, I have witnessed the power of these simple truths in action in his life and in the life of my patients when practiced. I hope every person who has the opportunity to read this book will incorporate them into their lives. Over time, the power of these practices to transform and heal are miraculous.

Michael has captured simplicity on the other side of the complexity of how the body, mind, and spirit must align to discover the "why" which connects us with the "who" that gives us the perseverance to learn the "how" to create new habits needed to overcome life's challenges.

Each person's journey is unique and, armed with these truths, will unfold to fulfill the purpose the Creator instilled within: not one of limitation, disability, and disease, but one of significance, lived with vitality, joy, kindness, self-control, patience, peace, and love.

– Scott Conard, MD DABFM, FAAFP, DABHIM / Converging Health & GOH Medical Dallas, Texas

Introduction

These 10 habits of wellness you are reading about were born out of need, extreme need! It began with excruciating pain that stabbed into my upper left chest with burning, biting intensity.

I knew I was having a heart attack!

As the pain radiated down my left arm and across my chest, I remembered my grandfather who had died at age 41. He had been on a hunting trip, told a joke, threw his head back in laughter, and dropped dead. My father had been diagnosed with heart disease around age 40 and his physician recommended a quadruple bypass. I had just turned 50, and with my family history, it seemed I was well overdue!

On the other hand, I had been a fitness buff since my teens and believed it would keep my heart healthy. I happened to be running up Troon Mountain in Arizona when the pain struck.

As I stood still on the mountain trail, hoping that, somehow, I might be able to get home before I died, my mind raced. How could this be happening to me?

Physically speaking, I was in good shape. I kept my weight in balance and I worked out. In fact, I often ran 25 to 30 miles in a week.

Spiritually, I felt strongly directed in my life's purpose. In my early twenties, I had gone to the jungles of Sumatra in Indonesia to work among the Batak tribe, known then as fierce head-hunters. I not only survived with my head intact but was adopted as a son by the chief. I had returned home to build a company to help non-profit organizations worldwide.

Emotionally and mentally, I was fully engaged. I had incredible drive and energy. I was focused, determined, and disciplined in everything I did.

Despite all that, I was the one having a heart attack!

I walked home slowly, thankful with every step that I was still alive. By the time I arrived, the pain had subsided. I convinced myself I didn't need to see a physician. It must have been an anomaly, I reasoned, because I was healthy and fit. And who wants to admit to having heart problems anyway!

> Many of us wait until, out of extreme need, we are forced to change our habits. A tip to the wise … when that happens, embrace the new habits quickly!

But there was a nagging suspicion in the back of my mind warning me that I was not as well as I wanted to believe. I was forced to admit to myself that it was strange how every year, for 25 years, I always got the flu, no matter what I did to protect myself from it. Also, I frequently got colds, despite the fact that I lived in sunny, dry Arizona.

And while I was at it, I had to admit that I often felt symptoms of stress. Running and lifting weights were my de-stressors.

Unfortunately, the pain returned the next day when I tried to exercise. It came sooner and lasted longer. My symptoms went from bad to worse. My entire left side was constantly in pain, from head to toe.

On several occasions over the following weeks, the pain was so great that my wife called 911, sure that I required medical treatment. I even drove myself to a local hospital and sat in my car outside the emergency room just in case I needed help.

But I had a business to run and goals to accomplish. The pain was a huge waste of my time!

When I finally went to a doctor, he said there was nothing wrong with my heart. But no answer was not helping, so I checked myself into Mayo Clinic to be examined for heart disease.

I went through their exhaustive series of examinations, beginning with heart tests, and they too found nothing wrong with my heart.

Soon after, I started having periodic "jolts," as if I had stuck my finger in an electrical outlet. These jolts started coming more and more frequently until I was having them about every ten minutes.

Back at Mayo Clinic, running a few more tests confirmed that I was cancer-free and having no respiratory problems. But they did find something wrong with my nervous system.

When I met with the physician, he told me, "You have a nervous system similar to a soldier who has been in a heavy-fire war for 30 straight years without a break. Your adrenal gland has produced adrenaline nearly nonstop and it has worn itself out. Your nervous system can no longer respond to any kind of pressure or emergency, not even a very slight symptom of physical or emotional stress."

In other words, my nervous system was toast! And the inflammation, the "jolts," and feeling like I was having regular heart attacks were the direct results.

The diagnosis brought a certain amount of relief, as I was grateful it wasn't heart disease or cancer, but the doctor explained, "There's nothing we can do for you. We have no cure, medication, surgery, physical therapy, or treatment that will give you a quick recovery."

A heavy-duty pain medication was an option, but it would do nothing to actually help my adrenal gland or nervous system repair itself. They said that it would take years before my nervous system could recover and respond to adrenaline without producing such incredible pain.

Their advice was to go home, sell my business or greatly scale back my involvement in it, relax, and be patient.

Being a results-oriented guy not known for his patience, this advice was not well received!

The Crux of the Matter

As part of the Mayo Clinic experience, it was recommended that I do a lifestyle study with one of their psychiatrists. How could talking to a shrink help my heart? Let's just say I was very skeptical!

At our meeting, the young psychiatrist thumbed through the pages of my report and asked, "Is this a true reflection of your lifestyle?"

"Yes, I guess," I replied. I had filled in the questionnaire as honestly and completely as I could.

When he started talking, it was one of those moments where time seemed to stand still. Everything around me blurred out as his words went straight to my heart, mind, and soul.

> Which is stronger, a copied behavior or a personal habit?

"You may think, Mr. Ellison, that you're out to save the world, but you are not Jesus Christ," he began. "And furthermore, when you die prematurely, your death will be noticed throughout the world like a pebble of sand thrown into the ocean. Nobody will celebrate your death 2,000 years later."

I didn't know what to say. I didn't like what he had said, but I knew it was the truth. And I was desperate for answers.

"I can't imagine how your wife has lived with you," he continued. "I can't imagine how your children could have lived with you all these years. For that matter, I can't even imagine how your employees in your company have worked for you. If you don't change the way you think about life, health, and work, you will die a premature death. And if you don't change the way you think, the quality of your life between now and the day you die will only get worse."

He put the matter of my health squarely into my hands. There was a very small glimmer of hope, but it depended solely on me changing. The trouble was I didn't know what to do differently! I wasn't even sure what was wrong about the way I had been thinking.

Yes, I knew I needed to change. It was a necessity. But what exactly did that mean? I was in great pain, lacked energy, and had an inflamed nervous system. My life was a mess. I had to find answers!

Unfortunately, I didn't have the foggiest idea where to begin.

When I got home, I stretched out on the floor and prayed. I pleaded, "God, please heal me so I can do the things that I believe You want me to do, do the things that I want to do, and be the kind of person that others want me to be."

No miraculous healing came. Instead, I really felt like God spoke to me, saying to my heart and mind, "No, Michael, I won't heal you. Don't even ask me for that. You do not understand wellness. If I heal you miraculously and instantly, you will only go back and abuse yourself again."

Everyone, God included, seemed to be in total agreement with the psychiatrist at the Mayo Clinic! Talk about ganging up on me!

I knew God would not do my thinking for me. He expected me to think and change. He expected me to seek and find a better way of living. He expected me to ask questions until I got answers.

When I got up from the floor, I was just as sick as before, but my attitude and perspective had changed.

I was a passionate seeker of wellness, and from that moment on, I have been on a journey to learn what it means to live life from that perspective.

Searching for Answers

As I started my personal search for wellness, I consulted the book that I have consulted throughout my life as a source of wisdom and counsel: the Bible. I found myself reading a verse of Scripture that I had read many times before, but on this particular day, it seemed to be in bold letters about two inches high: *"Do you not know that your body is the temple of the Holy Spirit, who you have from God, and you are not your own?"* (1 Corinthians 6:19, NKJV).

I put down my Bible and pinched the flesh on my arm and said out loud, "You are God's temple, Michael. You are here to glorify God in this temple."

Almost immediately, I added, "I will honor, I will nurture, and I will respect this temple God has given to me."

> If you don't live a NEW way of greater wellness, you are likely to die in your OLD ways.

Did I know how I would honor, nurture, and respect my body or my entire being in that moment? No, not at all. What I did do in that moment was change the way I saw myself. I changed the way I valued my "being," which included valuing my "body." I changed what I believed about my physical person.

Out of my change in belief, I made a commitment to learn how to honor, nurture, and respect the temple in which I dwelled, physically, emotionally, and spiritually.

Up until that moment, I hadn't really valued my physical body at all. My body simply was here and it did what my mind and emotions told it to do.

Suddenly, I saw my physical self in a whole new light. I saw myself as an intricate creation of God, designed for beauty and function as a reflection of God's awesome power and love.

I have always enjoyed the amazing beauty of nature, but never once did I stop to consider the fact that I was a creative work of nature myself. In that moment, I

Do We Have Genuine Wellness?

- We have so many food choices, yet so many empty calories, dangerous substances, and unhealthy ingredients in what we eat and drink.
- We have so many people around us at all times, yet so few genuine friends.
- We have so much entertainment, yet so little that is morally uplifting and inspirational.
- We have so much information available to us, yet so little is truly useful or important.
- We have so much stimuli that it is difficult to remember what we truly believe or value.

Stop and consider what you truly believe about your body, your wellness, and your purpose ... because what you believe is what you make into a habit.

grasped a new understanding that I was a creation of God, fearfully and wonderfully made. God intended for me to express Him on this earth through my physical being.

Certainly, I saw my work and accomplishments as a way of expressing God to the world around me, but that my physical body could be an expression as well? That was new to me.

But isn't that pride and arrogance?

I'd considered that, but I knew if my body was to express God's creation and love to the world, then I had to take my flesh seriously. After all, was my body not a "temple," and was I not responsible for it?

Clearly, this was going to require intentional effort. I was going to have to rethink how I valued myself.

In all likelihood, if you want to be serious about seeking wellness and embarking on a journey that leads to greater health and well-being, you will have to change the way you value yourself. You must believe as never before that:

- Your existence on this earth is important.
- You have a higher purpose and meaning than you've ever thought before.
- The care of your fleshly "temple" is worth the time and effort.

If these truths were going to become a reality in my life, then I was going to have to come up with habits that I could live with for the rest of my life. It would have to work, not once, but all of the time, and it would have to work physically, emotionally, and spiritually.

I didn't want easy, I wanted real. My future habits needed to work, be practical, and get repeatable results.

So began my life-changing journey to wellness.

The Help of Habits Along the Way

To achieve the wellness, health, and life that I wanted, I knew I needed help. That help came in the form of new, good habits.

It is easy to underestimate the power of making small improvements on a daily basis. People often look for a big "aha" moment to change everything, but rarely does that happen. Astonishing change occurs over time as we consistently use little incremental habits of wellness.

Yes, the habits may seem insignificant, but the impact can be exponentially huge! Sadly, few people use this to their advantage. How many people do you know who are wealthy after 40 years of saving money? (A single penny doubled 30 times results in more than five million dollars!) Accumulating debt is far more common, but it's the same process of taking small steps in any direction.

Good habits of wellness compound over time, just like money! And *that* is what I wanted. I knew the results would not be immediate, but they would be inevitable if I stuck with it. Trust me when I say that small habits

Make Habit #__ a Habit:

When you have a ***reminder*** of what you want, create a ***routine*** of doing what you want, and have a ***reward*** for getting what you want … you have a habit! You also get what you want!

#1: My reminder is …

#2: My routine is …

#3: My reward is …

of wellness over 5 or 10 years can be amazingly effective! I already knew the reverse was equally true.

What I learned about creating wellness habits I now call the "3 Rs" and they will make your wellness journey much easier.

Let me explain the 3 Rs:

> Habits form when we have 1) *reminders* in place that push us into an already-established 2) *routine*, which give us the 3) *rewards* we want.

There is a place in each chapter where you can take specific action toward the habits you want. You can write down your own reminder, routine, and reward.

And when you have made what you want a habit, you are on your way to getting it that much faster!

Habit #1

Sleep Peacefully

The reason for the habit?

– to rejuvenate your body and emotions so you are ready for each new day

Before I started on my journey of wellness, I had no regard for sleep, literally none whatsoever! I viewed sleep as an utter and complete waste of time, except on those occasional nights when I fell into bed completely exhausted. This occurred several times a year. I thought people who spent more than four hours sleeping in any given 24-hour period were lazy, poor managers of time, and not living up to their potential.

For decades, I slept three hours or less per night. I considered it an accomplishment to work through the night. It was a desirable goal for any given day. I was a driven man and I saw no reason to stop. Also, the company I founded was important to me. Seeing it grow and seeing more clients added to the company from around the world gave me personal satisfaction. I believed I was performing at my highest level.

But, in the end, I suffered physically and emotionally from this terrible habit. Lack of sleep is what caused most of the problems and inflammation in my nervous system, which drove me to the brink of disability and pre-mature death.

What I thought was a sign of efficiency, stewardship, and smarts was really an incredibly destructive habit based on my own faulty thinking. It was this thinking that sent me into my downward spiral.

I don't know about you and your view of sleep, but how you think about sleep impacts your overall health in many different ways. Consider for just a moment these insightful words from Ralph Waldo Emerson:

> "Sow a thought and you reap an action; sow an act and you reap a habit; sow a habit and you reap a character; sow a character and you reap a destiny."

One of the biggest breakthroughs for me related to this habit of sleep deprivation was learning just how beneficial sleep was to my health.

I had to change my thinking. If sleep was indeed good for me, and I knew I wanted to live and not die from my bad habits, then it only followed that I needed to ditch my ridiculous 3-hour sleeping habit!

> Make it your goal to create the habit of sleeping 7 to 9 hours a night.

For most people, changing habits begins with a change in how they think. That certainly was true in my case. I was forced to admit to myself that I didn't actually want the destiny I had sowed.

The change began when I decided I wanted the many benefits of sleep in my own life, including:

- A rejuvenated body

- Cells in my body being replenished and replaced
- Growth and development hormones being secreted properly
- Lower blood pressure
- Regaining energy
- The restoration and repair of major organs
- Restoration of damaged cells
- Memory consolidation

How could you not want those benefits in your life? I have no idea why I never let these blatant facts affect my actions. I should have embraced a good night's sleep many years ago. It would have saved me so much grief.

What was my excuse? I think I was too busy to pause long enough to think through the obvious.

How Much Sleep Do You Need?

Peaceful sleep is one of God's greatest gifts to our bodies. From a health standpoint, sleep is vital. Unfortunately, most people need more of it. Sleep deprivation has become a major disorder in our society, and this lack of sleep is contributing to our overall lack of wellness.

How much sleep do you need? Did you know that many professional athletes try to get 10 to 12 hours of sleep each night? That seems like a lot, but it only makes sense. When we sleep is when our bodies repair the most. This is true for the effects of physical exertion as well as the effects of stress on our bodies.

If you want your body to stay in optimal performance mode, make sure you get enough sleep for that to be a reality. Why would entire sports teams hire sleep experts to help the players unless it actually paid off?

Remember this simple truth:

> You can't fool your body.

In other words, get the sleep you need. Sleep experts say most adults need between 7 to 9 hours of sleep every night for optimum performance, health, rejuvenation, and safety. Teens need 8 to 9 hours.

A lot of people believe they can cut back on sleep during the week and make up for it on weekends, but if you stop and do the math, you'll quickly realize how improbable that is. For example:

> Let's say you only get 6 hours of sleep a night but need 7 to 9 hours. Using the middle ground (8 hours of sleep needed each week night), that means you are 12 hours short on sleep by the time you reach the weekend. Are you really going to take 6-hour naps on Saturday and Sunday afternoons to catch up?

That is a never-ending cycle that slowly hurts your body.

It is commonly reported that you need less sleep as you age. I consider this to be a myth. While aging may affect sleep patterns, it generally does not affect the amount of sleep your body needs. Older adults' bodies still need 7-9 hours each night. To reap the health benefits from good sleep, we all – regardless of age – need to aim for 7-9 hours of sleep each night.

Another myth is that it doesn't matter how long you sleep, only that you get a little bit of "deep sleep." When we sleep, we typically drift between 2 sleep states in 90-minute cycles.

Staying up all night is not good for your brain.
(*all-nighter)

For maximum rest and restoration, we all need at least 5-6 complete cycles of sleep a night. That means our bodies actually need 7-9 hours each night.

The Impact of Impaired Sleep

If ever the compound effect of sleep deprivation becomes a reality in our lives, it occurs when we keep going and going and going without sufficient sleep. The impact can be felt on many levels.

Physically, lack of sleep has a long list of negative results. Here are just a few:

- Impaired ability to use insulin, which can lead to the onset of diabetes
- Interruption of blood pressure cycles, which can lead to hypertension (high blood pressure) and cardiovascular problems
- Insufficient growth hormone secretion, which has been linked to obesity
- Impaired immunity, which can lead to greater susceptibility to disease

- Weight gain

Emotionally, lack of sleep has been correlated to:

- Increased anxiety, anger, and depression
- Difficulty controlling emotions

Mentally, some of the side effects from lack of sleep include:

- Difficulty concentrating or paying attention
- Difficulty remembering
- Decreased hand-eye coordination and other slowed responses

Financially, lack of sleep has a huge price tag. Not many people recognize the financial impact, but business owners certainly do. Consider these facts:

- Sleep deprivation and sleep disorders cost Americans an estimated $100 billion a year in lost productivity, medical expenses, sick leave, and property and environmental damage.
- Each year, tens of thousands of automobile crashes are caused by drowsy drivers, resulting in over 1,500 fatalities and many thousands of injuries. (*drowsy)

Unfortunately, living in a constant state of sleep deprivation is considered "normal" because most people are running on too little sleep. Of course, sleep deprivation is more extreme for those who have a chronic sleep disorder (which affects an estimated 40 million people), but it is estimated that 70 million people in the United States have some sort of sleep problem. That's a lot of people!

Nobody wants any of those symptoms!

Common Sleep Disorders

Sleep disorders are surprisingly common. Here are 7 to remember:

Plan your family's schedule so that each member of your family gets the sleep necessary to promote wellness.

1. **Sleep Apnea:** This is a breathing disorder where people have brief breathing interruptions all night long. They awaken frequently, sometimes gasping for breath. The pauses in breathing reduce the flow of blood oxygen to the brain, which is not good for the heart, brain, cardiovascular system, or metabolism. Obesity contributes to sleep apnea, and the increasing obesity rates are also increasing the occurrence of sleep apnea. Besides gasping for breath, another sign of sleep apnea is snoring on a frequent or regular basis, especially in irregular patterns. The good news is that sleep apnea can be treated, so if you think you might have this disorder (or think your spouse might have it), consult a physician.

2. **Restless Leg Syndrome:** This is a sleep and movement disorder characterized by tingling, crawling, creeping, or pulling feelings in the leg. People with this disorder have an overwhelming urge to move their legs to relieve the symptoms. This often results in almost constant kicking and shifting at night.

3. **Narcolepsy:** Talk about a dangerous disorder! Those who suffer from narcolepsy can suddenly experience a "sleep attack" at any time, day or night. Imagine sitting at a red light in busy traffic and suddenly you fall asleep at the wheel. I knew a man who had to put his car in park at red lights just in case he fell asleep suddenly.

4. **Insomnia:** Almost everyone has heard of this disorder, but it is more than just having trouble falling asleep. It is characterized by three distinct challenges: difficulty going to sleep, difficulty staying asleep, and waking up too early. Combine these three together and you have a very tired person in the morning! Repeat that over and over, day in and day out, and it is no wonder why wellness is so difficult to attain. Insomnia can be a medical or

> Sleeping less than 6 hours a night for 2 weeks forces your body to function as if you've missed an entire night's sleep.
> (*groggy)

psychological problem. In most cases, insomnia can be successfully treated.

5. **Delayed Sleep Phase Syndrome:** Also called Circadian Rhythm Disorder, this sleep disorder occurs when our brain's "biological clock" is off schedule. Imagine not being able to fall asleep until 3 or 4 AM and then sleeping until noon! That makes going to school or work a very difficult task! Due to the disorder, the body is off cycle and simply cannot get into the right schedule. Consult your doctor if this applies to you. It is usually treatable.

6. **Sleepwalking:** Though often laughed at, this sleep disorder is nerve-wracking and incredibly dangerous. Just like its name, sleepwalking is characterized by getting up in the middle of the night, while fully asleep, and wandering around. It is most common in children and, quite interestingly, it tends to run in families. I have heard of people waking up and finding themselves many miles from home. If someone in your house sleepwalks, keep the doors and windows locked at night.

7. **Sleep Terrors:** Those who suffer from this sleep disorder often scream, fight, or thrash about wildly while sleeping, but have no memory of it the next day.

A wide variety of treatments are available, including medication, light therapy, hormone treatment, continuous positive airway pressure (CPAP) devices, and scheduled naps. For some, a change in eating patterns will level the blood sugar levels, which can also help improve sleep.

> Sleep helps you control your hunger hormones. If you are tired, your "I'm hungry" hormone (ghrelin) is elevated. When you are well rested, your "I'm full" hormone (leptin) is in control. Which do you want to rule your day? (*hungry)

Make It a Habit

For a lot of people, it takes real planning to get a good night's sleep. This is especially true for those who suffer from a sleep disorder. It is also true for those who travel extensively across time zones or internationally where so many other factors may affect your sleep.

Part of the reason planning is required is that it can take some effort to tap into your own natural circadian rhythms, which governs the release of vital hormones within your body and put your body to sleep.

What can you do to get a better night's sleep? Here are 10 proven ways to improve the quality of your sleep:

1. **Avoid caffeine.** Avoid caffeine within 10 hours of your bedtime.

2. **Avoid alcohol near bedtime.** Although alcohol is a sedative with calming attributes, it can also increase the number of times you wake up in the latter half of sleep.

3. **Exercise regularly.** People who spend a lot of energy during the day as a result of walking, physical exercise, working out, and other forms of activity usually fall asleep faster and sleep better through the night than those with a less active lifestyle. With that said, it is recommended that physical exercise, such as an evening workout routine, be finished at least 3 hours before bedtime. This helps the body slow down and be ready for sleep.

4. **Watch what you eat.** Spicy foods and tomato products are notorious for causing heartburn in many people. Whatever the cause of heartburn, it makes falling asleep more difficult and causes more middle-of-the-night discomfort. Also, avoid eating too much before bedtime, or going to bed hungry, as both are known to disrupt sleep. Simply put, bedtime is

Ask Yourself:

Why do I want peaceful sleep?

____

____

____

____

not the best time for your body to be digesting a meal.

5. **Give up nicotine.** There are no health benefits to nicotine and it has been linked to difficulty falling asleep, problems waking up, and an increase in nightmares. Nicotine comes in many different forms these days, with special marketing efforts to reach the younger, more "hip" generation, but nobody, regardless of age, should willingly sign up for sleep deprivation.

6. **Restrict liquid intake.** Have your last glass of water 60-90 minutes before going to bed. This applies to all liquids, including herbal teas. Drink too close to bedtime and you'll need to get up in the middle of the night to use the bathroom, and that can really mess up your sleep cycle.

Do you battle depression? It may be in part due to a lack of sleep!
(*depression)

7. **Establish a relaxing bedtime routine.** You need to do what relaxes you. If it's a hot bath, warm shower, or a good book, create a routine and keep it. Dimming the lights 30 minutes before going to bed or closing the curtains to create a darker environment can also help. Basically, you are sending a signal to your brain that you are approaching the time to sleep, and you are

sending the same signal to your brain, day after day. This purposeful programming will help both your brain and your body to relax.

8. **Put yourself on a schedule.** Set a time when you will go to bed and when you will wake up. Then, do your best to make your daily routine match that set schedule. That means you will need to have completed any take-home work a few hours before bedtime and children should have their homework completed a couple hours before bedtime as well. This also applies to extracurricular activities, such as sports, parties, movies, and events. Any physical or mental activity needs to end well in advance of your predetermined bedtime. That includes internet surfing and computer games!

9. **Block out disruptive noise.** Use earplugs, create white noise, or play relaxing music to counteract disturbing noises, such as trains, sirens, loud conversations, airplanes, barking dogs, or early morning traffic. In some cases, you may choose to invest in rugs that absorb sound waves traveling through hard floors, hanging heavy curtains at your bedroom window, or installing double-paned windows. Blocking out disruptive noises also applies to any device in the bedroom (computers, pads, or phones), even if they give off the slightest noise.

10. **Get comfortable.** Create a sleep-friendly environment, one that includes a comfortable bed. I suggest keeping your bedroom dark, quiet, and slightly cool. Dark is important, so turn the clock away from your eyes. Do the same with any device that gives off light, even if the light is dim. You may want to purchase a humidifier or dehumidifier to regulate the humidity level. As for your bed, make sure your mattress provides the support you need. A good foundation or box spring is as important as a good mattress. If you search online, you will read descriptors about: breeze cooling systems, smart sleep technology, cooling, motion control, and support layers. It makes you want to jump in bed just to experience it! Also, check your pillow to make sure it provides adequate support for your neck. Check out my friend Mike Lindell, the "my-pillow man." He provides millions of people better quality of sleep with his designed pillows and mattresses. We both know the benefits of adding to your quality of life with a good night's sleep. If you use a body pillow, does it adequately support your arms and legs? Lastly, indulge a little in good quality bed linens. You will enjoy going to bed if your bedding is soft and luxurious. It will also

> If you aren't getting the sleep you need, go to bed 30 minutes earlier tonight. Keep backing it up until you are getting enough sleep.

improve your sleep, and that is the whole goal. Spending money for high quality sheets and pillow cases is worth it as you will spend up to a third of your life in bed! Don't be cheap about your sheets, pillows, mattress, or covers. There are countless great options today, so do your part to make sleeping inviting!

Don't feel pressured to try to apply all of these at once. I suggest doing one at a time. See if it helps. Then add another to your planning process. Step by step, your sleep will improve, and it will become a habit.

Make Sleeping Well a Habit:

When you have a ***reminder*** of what you want, create a ***routine*** of doing what you want, and have a ***reward*** for getting what you want … you have a habit! You also get what you want!

#1: My reminder is:

____

____

____

#2: My routine is:

____

____

____

#3: My reward is:

____

____

____

The more you value your sleep, the easier it is to make sure you are giving your body the amount of sleep it needs. All the benefits to your body a good night's rest brings make it entirely worth it!

Lastly, I recommend a simple prayer that has really helped me learn to sleep after decades of sleep deprivation. It goes like this:

> "Sleep, you are my friend. I invite you into my life to heal and rejuvenate my body. Thank you, God, for bringing sleep into my life."

I often had to say that prayer several times to myself before I fell asleep, but an amazing thing happened within two short weeks … I became a 7-hour-a-night sleeper!

For more than 30 years I deprived my body of the sleep it needed. That choice of mine was the foremost factor in my nervous system failure. It almost killed me! Thankfully, the new habit of getting enough sleep has played a huge part in the recovery of my nervous system.

If you know your body is not getting the amount of sleep it needs, choose to take action now.

Create this good habit now so that it can pay off to your advantage in the future.

Sleep does more than heal and rejuvenate our bodies. It can restore our sense of well-being, and that is a vitally important part of a vibrant and fulfilled life! We all want that.

Further Reading

*all-nighter: https://jamanetwork.com/journals/jamaneurology/fullarticle/1875833

*drowsy: https://one.nhtsa.gov/people/injury/drowsy_driving1/drowsy.html

*groggy: Van Dongen HP, Maislin G, Mullington JM, Dinges DF. The cumulative cost of additional wakefulness: dose-response effects on neurobehavioral functions and sleep physiology from chronic sleep restriction and total sleep deprivation. Sleep. 2003;26(2):117-126.

*hungry: https://www.nhlbi.nih.gov/node/4605

*depression: https://academic.oup.com/sleep/article/37/2/351/2558968

Habit #2

Breathe Deeply

The reason for the habit?

– to eliminate toxins, improve physical function, and decrease stress

One of the best things you can do to increase wellness is something you already do: breathe! Now, it is time to decide that you will breathe in a way that enhances your pursuit of wellness.

Good lung capacity and function are actually a vital part of your overall health. The average person, however, has a decline of lung capacity of 9-22% every decade! To combat that decline, maintain your lung capacity, because the greater your lung capacity, the longer you are likely to live.

Richard was someone who learned this out of necessity. For most of his life, he refused to do cardio exercises. To him, cardio exercise was unnecessary as he was strong in his upper body and preferred strength training. But when he went to the hospital for heart surgery, one of the first things the doctors explained was that his body needed more oxygen to ward off infection, such as pneumonia, and speed up his healing process. Suddenly, deep breathing was vitally important to him because it directly affected his ability to stay alive!

The good news is that we can all maintain and improve lung function through deep breathing techniques. Deep breathing, called "diaphragmatic breathing" by some, includes:

> Contraction of the diaphragm, expansion of the belly, and deepening of inhalation and exhalation, which consequently decreases the respiration frequency and maximizes the amount of blood gases. (*deep breathing)

10 Benefits of Good Lung Function

There are a lot of facts about lung function that most of us never learn. Here are 10 that may surprise you:

1. **Deep breathing of pure air removes toxins from the physical body.** The majority of the toxins we take into our bodies come through our lungs. We breathe in pollution in many forms (exhaust fumes, cigarette smoke, hairspray, allergens, etc.), but breathing also purges the body of 75% of the toxins we tend to ingest.

2. **Deep breathing is good for the brain.** Oxygen is vital to brain function. Brain cells use oxygen as we focus, concentrate, and remember. The deeper you breathe pure air, the greater your mental clarity and creativity. Deep breathing enhances your cognitive functioning, which enables you to make better decisions and solve problems.

3. **Deep breathing and breath control have shown to produce remarkable physical results.** Simply by breathing better, you may be able to lower your blood pressure, end heart arrhythmias, improve digestion, and increase blood circulation. All of these factors can lead to greater overall health.

4. **Deep breathing can reduce anxiety.** Deep breathing is foundational to alleviating stress and dissipating anger, anxiety, frustration, and impatience. Deep-breathing techniques have been shown to help people kick addictive and anti-anxiety drugs; it even helps treat PTSD. (*PTSD)

5. **Deep breathing improves your lymphatic system.** The health of your white blood cells, and your body's overall resistance to disease, is improved with deep breathing.

6. **Deep breathing gives you energy.** When you improve your bodily systems with deep breathing, it can, in turn, reduce anxiety, invigorate brain activity, and increase your overall energy.

Spirometer: a device that measures the volume of your inhaled and exhaled air. Expect a spirometry test if you are going in for surgery or if your lung function is in question.

7. **Deep breathing specifically helps women during critical stages of life.** Deep breathing and other breathing techniques have been shown to help women during pregnancy, increase the possibility of infertile women becoming pregnant, and reduce the frequency and intensity of hot flashes during menopause.

8. **Deep breathing can reduce pain.** Constant pain, common with diseases or injury, can be better managed with proper breathing.

9. **Deep breathing improves sleep quality and helps you fall asleep faster.** For me, sleep deprivation became a serious health problem. Learning to deep breathe before going to bed, and in the night when I woke up, significantly improved my sleep. The habit has brought the health benefits that come from sleeping longer and sleeping better. That is a longer life for me!

Learn how to breathe deeply.

10. **Deep breathing increases your oxygen intake.** Oxygen is a source of life, health, and well-being. The habit of deep breathing naturally increases your intake of oxygen in your blood, which in turn boosts oxygen and nutrient delivery to your cells. This is excellent news for your body's overall health.

In sum, by learning to breathe deeper, which is far better than shallow breathing, your level of wellness can directly improve.

Make the Choice to Breathe Pure Air

You may not be able to move to the country or to another city with a better climate and cleaner air, but there are things you can do to help create a less polluted personal space wherever you live, sleep, eat, and work. That can include:

- Putting fewer harmful chemicals onto your body, such as those often found in deodorants, skin care sprays, bug repellants, sunscreen lotions, and hairspray
- Spraying fewer harmful chemicals in your home, such as many found in cleaning and deodorizing agents or bug sprays
- Using fewer harmful chemicals in your garden or yard, such as those used to eliminate weeds and insects or to enhance the growth of flowers, fruits, or vegetables
- Avoiding smoke-filled environments and refusing to create a smoke-filled environment with cigarettes, cigars, or pipes
- Exercising caution with inhalants, gasoline fumes, paints, stains, and even fingernail polish
- Regularly replacing the air-conditioning or heating system air filters in your home

These are small steps, but they add up to you breathing purer air. You can also purchase an air purifier to help create a home atmosphere with cleaner air.

Practice Breathing Like a Baby

A baby automatically breathes abdominally with their diaphragm (the muscles just at the base of the rib cage), but most adults use only their chest muscles to breathe. This shallow breathing or chest breathing only pulls in a minimal amount of air into the lungs. Most people who shallow breathe are not aware that they do it.

Several conditions may contribute to shallow breathing, such as anxiety disorders, asthma, pulmonary edema, panic attacks, stress, or just all-around anxiousness about life.

> Slow, controlled breathing has been found to increase longevity.
> (*live longer)

Only when you compare deep breathing to shallow breathing do you see how much you have been missing.

Practice using your diaphragm.

If you have never consciously breathed in this fashion, you can learn "deep breathing" techniques. Here is how:

> Lie on your back and put one hand on your upper abdomen and one hand on your upper chest. As you inhale, try to raise the hand on your abdomen with your breath. Think of it as if you are trying to inflate your belly, not your

> lungs. As you exhale, push down with your hand on your abdomen as if gently forcing the air out of your lungs.

Repeat this technique until you can tell that you are pushing air out of your lungs by using your diaphragm and allowing air into your lungs by relaxing the diaphragm. It may take a little practice!

Here is another good description of the deep breathing:

> Close your mouth and inhale through your nose for a count of 4. Hold your breath for a count of 7, then exhale through your mouth making a "whoosh" sound. If you cannot do this when starting to form your breathing habit, then use a 2 and 4 count ratio until you can work up to the 4 and 7.

The best times each day to practice deep breathing include:

- When you wake up
- Before you go to sleep
- When you wake up in the middle of the night
- Mid-morning and mid-afternoon
- Any time you need to decrease stress (i.e. during a long commute)

Additional Benefits of Deep Breathing

Deep breathing has even been shown to help people let go of harmful emotions. Similarly, did you know that many negative emotions are linked directly to our breathing patterns? For example:

- Anger is commonly associated with shallow inhalation, strong exhalation, and increased muscle tension throughout the body, especially the neck, jaw, chest, and hands.
- Fear is associated with rapid, shallow, and irregular breathing, as well as a tightened "knot" in the lower abdomen.
- Grief and sorrow are associated with spasmodic, sobbing, superficial breathing, and a hollow feeling in the abdomen.
- Impatience has been associated with short, jerky, uncoordinated breathing and tension in the front of the chest.
- Guilt or self-judgment has been linked to restricted, suffocating breathing and an overall sensation of being weighed down.
- Boredom has been associated with shallow, lifeless breath and little sensation anywhere in the body.

Ask Yourself:

Why do I want to breathe deeply?

____

____

____

____

It is interesting to note that all of these negative emotions are linked to shallow, constricted, or faulty breathing.

On the other hand, deep breathing can reverse these emotions, especially when accompanied by relaxation techniques. Studies have shown that deep, comfortable breathing is associated with feelings of openness, energy, and positive emotions, such as love, compassion, kindness, and awe.

Deep breathing has also been linked to greater creativity and improved self-image. This certainly makes sense, as pure air is linked to wellness and greater mental clarity.

Deep breathing 7x a day can greatly increase the efficiency of your immune system. (*immune)

Make It a Habit

One of the best ways to create this new habit is to practice doing it while you are busy with something else. For example, if you are watching TV, riding in a car, or reading a book, you can practice deep breathing.

In the context of the habit loop of the 3 Rs (Reminder, Routine, and Rewards), you know the reward. Suppose watching TV is the routine. How then could you establish a reminder when watching TV to practice your deep breathing? Perhaps you could leave this book on a table near the TV as your reminder? Or maybe put a note by the remote control with "BREATHE!" in big letters? Make your own reminder to remember. Then you are on your way to establishing your habit!

Naturally, the more you practice deep breathing, the better you get at it, and the closer and closer it moves to becoming a full-blown habit. That is what you want.

We all need clear thinking and mental energy. Deep breathing can help.

Once you have learned to breathe abdominally with your diaphragm, take "breathing breaks" during the day. Start with just a couple minutes twice a day, but try to work up to 10 minutes a day. Take at least two 10-minute breathing breaks each day, and a third breathing break just before going to sleep.

As you engage in deep breathing:

> Close your eyes and keep your back straight. Begin with a deep, audible sigh, then quietly inhale. See how slow, deep, and regular you can make your breathing. You should constantly feel as if you are getting enough air. Do this for at least 8 deep breaths, then open your eyes and breathe normally.

There are several variations of deep breathing. At times, focus on inhaling and make it as long as possible. Breathe in through your nostrils and exhale through your mouth. Other times, focus on exhaling more than inhaling. Attempt to squeeze all the air out of your lungs. You should be able to feel the muscles that help do this.

Make Breathing Deeply a Habit:

When you have a ***reminder*** of what you want, create a ***routine*** of doing what you want, and have a ***reward*** for getting what you want ... you have a habit! You also get what you want!

#1: My reminder is:

____

____

____

#2: My routine is:

____

____

____

#3: My reward is:

____

____

____

Do not be concerned if you feel a little lightheaded as you first begin to breathe deeply. This will pass as you become more accustomed to breathing from the belly.

Regular deep breathing improves your overall lung capacity, and that directly benefits you in many different ways. It is a vital part of your overall wellness.

...

As you practice deep breathing, see yourself as inhaling the wonderment of creation, faith, hope, love, and all things good.

Exhale completely. As you do, exhale your problems, fears, anxieties, frustrations, stress, and all things negative.

You might want to take a deep breathing break right now!

Further Reading

*deep breathing: https://www.ncbi.nlm.nih.gov/pmc/articles/pmc5455070/)

*PTSD: https://academic.oup.com/jcem/article-abstract/98/7/2984/2537196

*live longer: Radaelli A, Raco R, Perfetti PI, et al. Effects of slow, controlled breathing on baroreceptor control of heart rate and blood pressure in healthy men. J Hypertens 2004; 22: 1361-1370.

*immune: http://options4fitness.com/options-4-relaxation/how-deep-breathing-can-help-improve-your-immune-system/

Habit #3

Drink Pure Water

The reason for the habit?

– to create greater health, look younger, and feel better

Are you a water drinker? Before I started on my journey toward wellness, I drank coffee, iced tea, and soft drinks (energy drinks). That was it! And if it didn't have sugar and caffeine, I didn't drink it. "Why drink water?" I reasoned, "It has no taste. It doesn't give me any extra energy. It does nothing to help my intense performance-driven lifestyle."

But water, as I learned on my wellness journey, is a critical part of good health. Nothing hydrates the body like water, and few things do more to promote health than drinking pure water in sufficient quantity. And truth be told, it does indeed enhance your energy!

I did not think water did anything to give me energy, but almost immediately after I made water my beverage of choice, I noticed a real increase in my mental and physical energy without the spikes and lows of stimulants.

Since then, I have heard hundreds of people say the very same thing. In fact, years ago, I went on a week-long wilderness adventure with an outfitter and several guides who only drank sodas and energy drinks. I offered them a challenge: change to water and see if their energy levels remain higher all day. By the time the week was up, water was the beverage of choice!

Water not only adds energy, it is far better at supporting every system and organ in your body than soda and energy drinks.

Next to oxygen, water is the most critical substance for life. It has been called the "silent nutrient" for wellness, a "must have" for life. Even Henry David Thoreau wrote:

"Water is the only drink for a wise man."

Your body may appear to be more solid than fluid, but in actual fact, your body is 60% water as an adult. Water comprises most of your body's fluids, including your blood.

Every single physical system in your body depends on sufficient water, and that includes respiration, circulation, digestion, brain function, joint function, energy production, and waste removal.

Drinking Water Helps You Lose Weight

Especially if you:

- Drink cold water (your body will spend energy heating it up)
- Drink water 30 minutes before meals (this makes you less hungry)
- Drink at least 9 cups per day (boosts your metabolism)

(*weight loss)

The water you routinely lose through perspiration, urination, bowel movements, and exhalation need to be replaced regularly and sufficiently so that you can maintain your physical health.

Refilling your body with the water it needs to function at its optimal level is what this is all about. It sounds simple enough, but you would be surprised how few people actually do this!

10 Benefits of Water

The benefits of drinking enough water so that you are sufficiently hydrated include:

1. Water regulates your body temperature.
2. Water lubricates your joints (knees, elbows, wrists, fingers, etc.). This means less joint pain and improved flexibility.
3. Water helps dissolve minerals and other nutrients so your body can put them to use.
4. Water helps prevent constipation.
5. Water carries nutrients and oxygen to all cells of the body, helping the whole body thrive.
6. Water moistens the tissues of the mouth, eyes, and nose.
7. Water lessons the burden on the kidneys and liver by flushing out waste products.
8. Water has a rejuvenating effect on our energy levels.

Does Drinking Water Cause Water Retention?

If your body is not sufficiently hydrated, it tends to hoard or retain water. This isn't fat, but it can be discouraging if you are trying to lose weight.

However, when your body has sufficient hydration, it releases the water. Toxins and waste materials, including fat, are more readily flushed from the system.

If water retention is a concern, make sure you are drinking enough water every day. It is easy to fix.

9. Water helps with weight loss and weight maintenance.
10. Water enhances your skin texture and appearance.

All of these physical benefits add up to a healthier you!

How Dehydration Affects You

The opposite of sufficient hydration, of course, is dehydration. This occurs when your body does not have enough water to carry out its normal functions.

Most people think that dehydration occurs only when they are extremely sick or if they happen to get lost in a desert. But the fact is, dehydration is incredibly common.

Here is a startling truth:

Most people are mildly dehydrated.

Very few people drink enough water every single day. Living mildly dehydrated can continue unnoticed for years because the body learns to cope with it as best it can. But coping is not thriving, and there are negative side effects, such as low energy levels, constant fatigue, feeling sluggish, and bloating.

How do you know if you are mildly dehydrated? Here are some of the most common symptoms, which tend to be more prominent in the very young or very old:

- Excessive thirst
- Fatigue
- Dry skin, mouth, and hair
- Asthma and allergies
- Headaches
- Muscle weakness
- Dizziness or lightheadedness
- Constipation
- Little or no urination
- Urine that is dark or cloudy
- Moodiness
- Lack of concentration
- Increased risk of kidney stones (*kidney)

These "mild" impairments from dehydration may pass off as normal, but why live with these problems if you don't have to? All you need to do is get in the habit of drinking more water.

More extreme results of dehydration include sunken eyes, fainting, rapid heart rate, dizziness, and seizures. Of course, nobody wants these health issues, but the distance between mildly dehydrated and dehydrated is not all that great.

When Your Body Uses the Most Water

Your body is constantly using water, which is why the need exists to constantly be refilling it. There are times, however, when our bodies use more water than normal. Being aware can help you be more prepared.

Peak water use in your body occurs at these times:

1. **In the bathroom.** Naturally, most of your water loss occurs when you use the bathroom.

2. **Sweating and breathing:** The next biggest water usage comes while sweating and breathing. The evaporation of water from your body, which happens day and night, is about a pint, which is 2 cups (16 oz) of water every day. (*evaporation)

3. **During exertion.** If you are engaging in any activity that results in perspiration, you need extra water to compensate for the fluid loss. To compensate for a short period of exercise, you need several cups of water. If you have a high-exertion job, such as hauling or lifting heavy objects all day, you need a lot more fluid at regular intervals. If the exertion involves

significant perspiration, you need to replace sodium as well as fluid. I remember a time when I was hiking the La Plata mountain range, which are very steep, with my son, Luke. He had worked hard to get in very good shape for this excursion. There were times he went off the trail ahead of me or out on a ridge point, just enjoying the best fitness of his life and the wonderful views in the mountains. But later that afternoon, something happened that could have been catastrophic. He had not been drinking enough water and he experienced extreme dehydration and an imbalance of electrolytes, all of which led him into semi-shock. Thirst is not an indicator of the amount of water needed during exertion. He learned to drink water during exertion, whether he felt thirsty or not.

> Technically speaking, sparkling water, seltzer, soda water, tonic water, and club soda are soft drinks. They should not count toward your daily water intake.

4. **When sick.** When you are sick, you need additional water to flush toxins and waste from the body. If fever, vomiting, or diarrhea come with the sickness, then it is especially critical to replace the lost fluids. Water with electrolytes may be necessary. People die every day due to severe dehydration.

Additives That Subtract:

Most beverages contain water, but it's the other ingredients that can harm your health. These additives include:

- *Sugar:* Juices often have high levels of added sugar, while sodas can have as much as 12 teaspoons of sugar per serving.
- *Fats:* Dairy products have some water, but also milk solids generally composed of fats that convert to sugar (lactose) in your body.
- *Caffeine:* As a stimulant, caffeine can trigger a slight increase in metabolism, but it can also trigger a craving for food.

5. **If pregnant or breast feeding.** It is recommended that pregnant women drink nearly 10 cups of water each day, while women who are breastfeeding should drink about 13 cups daily.

6. **In hot weather or high altitude.** It only makes sense that we need to drink more water in hot or humid weather because we are sweating more, but heated indoor air can also cause a loss of moisture. Even altitude plays a part. Higher than 8,200 feet above sea level, your

Additives That Subtract: (continued)

- ***Sodium:*** Most carbonated beverages have sodium (salt), as do soups (canned or dry). Your body needs some sodium, it must be balanced with potassium to reduce the risk of chronic disease. The typical North American diet is too high in salt and too low in potassium.
- ***Aspartame:*** Many drinks are sweetened with Aspartame, a chemical reportedly tied to unhealthy side effects and negative symptoms in the brain, body, and blood sugar levels.

Always make sure what you are drinking is pushing you closer to your wellness goals.

body needs more water. Higher altitudes can also trigger increased urination and more rapid breathing, which help burn up more of your body's fluid reserves. Did you know that the humidity on an aircraft is approximately the same as the humidity of the Sahara Desert? (*dry air) A long flight can be exhausting, even though all you did was just sit there. That is because your body thinks it is in a desert, so be sure to drink plenty of water on long trips, especially international flights.

7. **With certain foods.** Your body needs extra water if you are eating salty foods or are on a high protein diet. Consuming high fiber foods or supplements increases your need for water in order to keep your digestive tract working normally. As odd as it may seem, some beverages actually have a mild dehydrating effect because they trigger your body to release water, which makes it more of a challenge to maintain a healthy internal water balance. Drinks that do this to your body include caffeinated coffees, teas, sodas, and alcoholic beverages. The remedy for this is simple: for every cup of caffeinated or alcoholic beverage you drink, increase your water intake by one cup as well.

8. **When sleeping.** Getting 7.5-9 hours of sleep each night is recommended, but technically your body is dehydrating itself for those same hours! We don't usually think of sleep as being naturally dehydrating, but it is. First thing in the morning, be sure to drink sufficient water to get you hydrated again. I suggest at least 2 cups of water at that time.

How Much Water Do You Really Need?

We talk about drinking water, needing water, and making sure we get enough water each day, but just how much water are we supposed to drink?

The answer is pretty simple. It is based on your weight.

Here is the basic formula:

Step #1: Your weight (in lbs):

= _____

Step #2: Divide that by 2:

= _____

Step #3: That number divided by 8 (because there are 8 oz/cup):

= _____

ANSWER: The number you are left with is the number of cups of water you need to drink each day.

For example, if someone weighs 176 pounds, half of that is 88, which then becomes the number of fluid ounces of water the person needs every day. The 88, at 8 oz/cup, equals 11 cups of water. This coincides with the Institute of Medicine (IOM) and their average daily recommendation of 13 cups of water for men and 9 cups for women. (*water)

Is your water bottle made of non-leaching plastic?

Most people just assume they are getting enough water. Yes, there is water in the foods we eat (cucumbers are 95% water, celery is 90% water, and oranges are 87% water), but it is safer to only count the cups of water you drink. Studies have found that about 20% of our water intake comes from the foods we eat (*food water), but don't rely on it. I recommend that you just count it as a "bonus" and still drink your necessary glasses of water.

When it comes to calculating your actual water intake, don't assume anything. Most people are not drinking enough water and numerous surveys have shown that people routinely overestimate their water consumption. Figure your required water intake, and then follow through on that amount.

Test yourself:

> Fill a 32-ounce container with water and drink from it all day long. Drink water from no other source. You may be surprised at how much water you still have in the container by nightfall, and it's only 4 cups of water! You should go through two or three 32-ounce containers if you are getting sufficient water.

Remember, your body needs around 9-13 cups each day. If you are not getting that amount, you simply cannot get the best performance from your body. Fill up your glass of water and do it often!

Best Ways to Get "Pure" Water

Did you know that "bottled water," in many cases, is no safer or less contaminated than regular tap water?

If you buy bottles of water, check the bottle itself. Make sure it is made of non-leaching plastic, so the plastic is not releasing possibly harmful toxins into the water.

Non-leaching plastic bottles can generally be cleaned with pure hot water and reused.

To ensure that your water is pure, you need to make sure it has been filtered. Unfiltered water can carry toxins, parasites, and heavy metals. The jury is still out when it comes to the toxicity of fluoride and chlorine used in metropolitan water systems. Several long-range studies of these chemicals, which have been routinely added to some public water systems for decades, have yielded alarming results.

Also, if you live in an older home that has lead pipes, or even in a new home with copper pipes with lead soldering at the joints, you may want to have your water tested for toxins.

In order to purify or filter your own water, you need some type of water purification system. When considering such a system, understand these terms:

> ***Distillation*** is the process of turning water into vapor. As water vaporizes, the heavy metals are left behind. When the vapors are collected and condensed into water again, the water should be pure.

> ***Reverse osmosis*** is the process of forcing water through membranes to remove minerals in the water.

> ***Absolute 1-micron filtration*** uses filters that remove particles larger than one micron in

size, which tends to eliminate parasites as well as heavy metals.

Ozonation is not generally a home purifying technique, but one used by commercial bottlers. Ozone gas (an antimicrobial agent) is used to disinfect the water instead of using chlorine to do so.

Water treated by one of these four processes does meet the standards of "purified" water by the U.S. Pharmacopeia.

Recognize that every water purification and filtration system requires regular maintenance. Without proper maintenance, bacteria or other contaminants can build up.

I personally recommend water purification systems that serve all the faucets in the home, including bathtubs and showers.

Make It a Habit

Thirst is not a reliable gauge for when and how much you should drink. You need to hydrate your body

Ask Yourself:

Why do I want to drink pure water?

____

____

____

____

before your body demands it. Thirst is actually a warning signal. Your body is saying, "I NEED WATER!" Your body has no middle ground, no pre-warning system. When you are thirsty, your body really needs water, and right then!

A friend of mine really loves his coffee. Basically, he drinks coffee nonstop. Yes, coffee is liquid, but it is no replacement for water. Only water can support your body's systems and organs and help balance electrolytes in your body in the most efficient manner.

Our bodies can live and function to some degree while being dehydrated, but we cannot function very well long-term without good hydration.

> **Water Calculator**
>
> Your weight (in lbs): ____
>
> Divide by 2: ____
>
> Divide by 8: ____
>
> This number = the cups of water you need to drink each day.

My coffee-drinking friend and I were golfing with a few other golfing buddies one day when he suddenly began to feel weak and light headed. In just minutes he was so sick that we had to call 911 and he ended up in the hospital. And his diagnosis? It was dehydration!

None of us should use thirst as an indicator of our need for water consumption. Interestingly, older people sense thirst less, so regular hydration becomes more important as we age. Conversely, younger people tend to ignore the warning signs, which can cause troubles later on.

Whatever your age, make it a habit to stay hydrated. After all, it's your body, and all you need to do is hit the daily amount of water intake based on your body weight. It's simple!

Here are several ways to make hydration a habit:

1. **Drink first thing:** Drink a glass of water immediately upon arising in the morning and another one 30 minutes later. Since most glasses hold around 12 ounces, you will have taken in three cups of water in the first 30 minutes of your day. That's a good start!

2. **Drink before working out:** Drink 1 or 2 glasses of water 30-60 minutes before exercising. You know you're going to lose water during your workout, so prepare your body in advance.

3. **Keep it handy:** Always have a water bottle at your desk or in your car. Sip from it often or train yourself to drink at least one cup (8 oz) every hour during the day.

4. **Take water breaks:** These are better than coffee breaks, cigarette breaks, or donut breaks. Refill your water bottle or have a large glass of water during break time.

5. **Swap it out:** Choose a sparkling water at social gatherings rather than an alcoholic beverage. You'll feel better … and drive home safely!

6. **Add a twist:** A little lemon or lime juice in your water can add a nice burst of flavor. You'll find it especially refreshing in hot weather.

7. **Put ice on it:** Fill your water bottle to about an inch from the top and freeze it overnight. This will give you cold water for most of the day.

Make Drinking Pure Water a Habit:

When you have a ***reminder*** of what you want, create a ***routine*** of doing what you want, and have a ***reward*** for getting what you want … you have a habit! You also get what you want!

#1: My reminder is:

____

____

____

#2: My routine is:

____

____

____

#3: My reward is:

____

____

____

When you drink sufficient pure water, you have an emotional sense of satisfaction as you nourish your body for greater health. Pure cool water on a hot day is one of the most satisfying things I can imagine. Water refreshes, not only physically, but also emotionally, and that certainly helps with habit formation!

My wife, Susan, is a habitual water drinker. She created her own habit loop (Reminder, Routine, and Reward) to help her accomplish what she wants each day. Her goal is 60-80 ounces of water per day. Her routine is to get up in the morning and make a cup of coffee to drink while she has her morning meditation, prayer, and devotional readings. While the coffee is brewing, she pours a 32-ounce pitcher of water and places it on the kitchen counter as a reminder to drink from it all day long. When it's empty, she refills it.

By the end of the day, she has easily attained her 60-80 ounces of water.

One reward is her beautiful, hydrated skin. She has had many young women ask her what lotion she uses to have such beautiful skin. It's not lotion at all, it's water!

Thankfully, filling your body with sufficient pure water is one of the easiest things you can do to promote good health. Make it a habit and you are well on your way!

Further Reading

*weight loss: https://www.healthline.com/nutrition/7-health-benefits-of-water#section3

*kidney: https://www.webmd.com/diet/features/6-reasons-to-drink-water

*evaporation: http://extensionpubs.unl.edu/publication/900001 6361981/water/

*dry air: https://www.news.com.au/travel/travel-advice/flights/ flying-secrets-no-one-talks-about/news-story/632a8916be06c36 e39a24ea9f531e017

*water: https://www.healthline.com/health/how-much-water-should-I-drink

*food water: https://www.ncbi.nlm.nih.gov/pmc/articles/PMC 2908954/

Habit #4

Eat Nutritiously

The reason for the habit?

– to have a happy and healthy lifestyle with less illness and disease!

Many years ago, we had a five-year drought hit our ranch in southern Colorado. Soon after that, the pine bark beetles arrived and thousands of trees on the ranch and across parts of the state seemed to die overnight.

How could such a tiny insect produce such devastating results? It turned out that a weakness in the tree was a far bigger problem than the strength of the beetle.

Normally, when a pine bark beetle begins to drill through the bark of a pine tree, the tree produces sap that fills the hole and stops the intrusion. However, the drought-stricken trees had been deprived of key nutrients and could not secrete the necessary sap. They were defenseless as the beetles burrowed deep into the core, severing and disrupting the upward flow of water and nutrients at multiple points. The tree's lifelines were cut, and death came quickly.

The lesson is simple:

> The trees were malnourished and could do nothing to stop the invasive beetles.

But this life lesson also applies to human beings.

No, most people are not usually severely malnourished or doing anything particularly bad when it comes to the way they treat their bodies (they aren't intentionally starving themselves or drinking poison). They are, however, depriving themselves of the nutrients needed for good health by not eating a balance of nutrients to support their body's systems and organs. And if their bodies are not truly strong on the inside, are they not just like the drought-stricken trees? When disease or injury occurs, does the body have what it needs to defend, heal, and restore itself?

That is the question, and it is definitively answered when a crisis happens ... but that is NOT the time to find out if your body is prepared and strong enough!

This then is our goal:

> To eat a balanced diet that supports a healthy and happy lifestyle, so if disease or injury does occur, our bodies are better able to heal and restore our health.

Remember, your body is designed to heal itself. Your job is to explore and learn what best gives your body the right balance of nutrients and nurturing support.

Making the 10 habits of wellness actual habits in your life will do just that for your body, physically, emotionally, and spiritually. You will have greater energy, improved strength, and an overall sense of well-being, and that is your body's best defense!

It's also the best way to live life to the fullest here and now. You can live a happier and healthier lifestyle with less illness and disease, with greater vitality and energy, by embracing the habit of eating nutritiously. After all, that is the goal and reward of eating nutritiously.

Your Body Is Incredible!

What is amazing about the human body is that it was designed to both heal itself and resist disease. Again, I am reminded of Psalms 139:14, which says, *"I will praise You, for I am fearfully and wonderfully made. Marvelous are Your works!"* (NKJ). The built-in repair system of a healthy person constantly produces new cells to replace old, worn, or weakened cells, all while the immune system is constantly resisting disease. It is remarkable, truly awe-inspiring, in its design and effectiveness.

Eating nutritious food is great, but doing so *consistently* is the best way to defend against sickness.
(*consistent)

However, to function as designed, the body must first have the right fuel in its system. Without the right fuel, the body (just like the drought-stricken trees) won't be able to repair or resist disease. The pine beetle would not have been so successful in destroying the trees if the trees were healthy with the proper moisture and nutrients.

How many sicknesses, diseases, or accidents were more impactful, even deadly, than they should have been? We all hear of people going into the hospital for a common surgery and ending up getting pneumonia or some other life-threatening issue because their bodies were already in a weakened condition. Why is that? Because they did not have wellness habits in place before they went to the hospital!

What is one of the most common reasons for self-healing or not? For frequent sickness or not? It is this:

> What goes in your mouth will significantly determine how healthy your body will be.

That is the core message of staying healthy! It is the central reason for creating good eating habits. You must think about what you put into your mouth from this perspective, then choose to eat what your body needs for health.

It has been estimated that a mere single serving of fruits and vegetables taken daily will save trillions of dollars and tens of thousands of lives each and every year. (*veggies)

Yes, your body is incredible, but the choices you make on a daily basis (choosing to eat foods that are full of nutrients or void of nutrients) will determine how well your body will function. That is motivation!

When you know why your body needs the right fuel, it makes creating the right habit so much easier, doesn't it?

Making Food Choices on Purpose

For many years, I was fit and incredibly energetic. I worked out and ran regularly. It didn't seem to matter what I fed my body (steak, pasta, potatoes, pizza, soda, caffeine, or sugar), I ate in quantities that allowed me to maintain my weight. If I gained a pound or two, I simply worked out a little longer or harder to lose those pounds.

Admittedly, most of what I fed my body was more pleasing to my taste buds and my body's comforts than it was about setting my body up for success. I shudder to think what my real health was like at the cellular level.

In the aftermath of my nervous system inflammation that nearly stole my life, I realized how serious it was and now I intentionally feed my body the fuel it actually needs. I could no longer look to just satisfy my "wants," I had to look to meet my body's "needs."

So what do you eat or avoid eating if you are trying to give your body the fuel it needs to live happy and healthy with less illness and disease? In the next few pages, I offer four choices or guidelines for nutrition that you can apply to your life. These are not intended to be exhaustive lists of foods to eat or not eat. Rather, these guidelines will help you form your own eating habits that will give your body the nutrition that it needs. Maybe just as important to note is that if you follow these guidelines you will reduce the inflammatory effects of high glycemic foods, or foods filled with hormone enhancement, antibiotics, or pesticides.

One additional piece of the nutritious eating puzzle is the mindset of supporting your belief in who you are and why you matter. You matter and your choice of foods matter to your health! This belief will help you create and maintain your wellness habit of eating nutritiously.

These four food choice guidelines made a tremendous difference in my wellness journey. They include:

Choice #1 – Eat whole foods instead of processed foods. Make it your goal to avoid all processed foods, processed meats, and grains. This alone will greatly enhance your health.

Whole foods are those that can be plucked directly from a tree or pulled from a garden, such as fruits, vegetables, nuts, and seeds. These foods are best eaten fresh, raw, or lightly steamed. This includes whole grains, legumes, beans, and eggs. Eating organic is preferred because non-organic foods unfortunately have pesticides and other chemicals, which can cause an inflammatory response in your body. A word of caution here: there is significant research coming forward that too much grain is not healthy for your brain. Your brain needs healthy fats, not a high carb low fat diet. (I recommend the Bredesen Protocol as additional research, especially if know you carry the ApoE4 gene, which increases your risk of dementia and Alzheimer's.)

In comparison, processed foods include packaged foods, what you get at fast food restaurants and commercial bakeries, many frozen foods, chips and snacks, processed sandwich meats, and most canned foods.

The three big "processes" to avoid are:

1) Whole grains processed into white flour. The alternative is whole wheat or almond flour.
2) Cane or beets processed into white sugar, and that includes all artificial sweeteners. The alternative would be a natural sweetener like stevia.
3) Fats processed through hydrogenation. The alternative is ghee or mono-saturated fats.

When you eliminate white flour, white sugar, and hydrogenated fats (including trans fats and partially hydrogenated fats), every cell in your body and brain will thank you!

Processed foods are also usually loaded with salt, some form of bad fat, sugar, and chemical additives. When you read the label on any packaged or canned food item and cannot pronounce an ingredient, it is probably not good for you! Your body simply doesn't recognize it as food and generally will have an inflammatory reaction to it. When you make the change to eating more whole foods, food

Regulated or "even" blood sugar levels help your body avoid resorting to adrenaline to sustain energy or cope with stress. Feeding your body the right foods brings you the balance you need. Control the release of adrenaline and insulin into your body and you reduce the likelihood of developing diabetes.

may seem "bland." But this will change as your taste buds adjust.

When it comes to dairy products, I recommend grass-fed organic butter, milk, cottage cheese, or yogurt. You need the fat, calcium, and amino acids from dairy products. For those who are lactose intolerant, using nut milks is a good alternative. Everyone should avoid products laced with sugar or sugar-based flavoring, such as milkshakes and ice cream.

As you add more vegetables and fruit to your diet, try to choose organically grown produce because organically grown produce have not been treated with pesticides, fungicides, or chemicals that might detract from wellness. These substances can be inflammatory triggers as they are not identified by your body as foods and your body will respond as if they are foreign invaders. Inflammation, and all the symptoms that come with it, is the natural result.

The increase in whole vegetables and fruits will likely increase your intake of fiber, which is great. Fiber can "scrub clean" the walls of the intestines and colon, freeing your body of fatty build-up that inhibits the absorption of nutrients into the blood stream.

Countries that typically eat whole foods, but that have shifted to more processed foods, are now experiencing dramatic increases in their obesity rates. (*obesity) Why the sudden and alarming increase in obesity among children and adults? It happens everywhere and is simply the result of eating foods that have little nutritional value but contain dense calories.

Choice #2 – Eat lean meats. Choose to eat more lean meats, like fish, chicken, and turkey, and less red meat (unless it is certified grass-fed). A lot of research and studies strongly support grass-fed red meat as being healthy. Always grill, bake, or broil rather than fry. If frying, try using ghee or avocado oil (because these have a high heat smoke point) and olive oil for medium heat (best for sautéing).

Red meat, including ground meat, generally contains high amounts of fat in which toxins are absorbed and accumulated (if not organically grass-fed). If you do eat red meat, select the leanest cuts possible. Also, choose range-fed meats as they have less antibiotics or genetically engineered substances than regular production feedlot meats.

With fish, you want fish high in omega-3 fatty acids, such as salmon, cod, albacore tuna, haddock, bluefish, and sardines. Buy wild-caught whenever possible. True cod is one of the most reasonably priced and best light fish you can buy (Try a sautéed approach with olive oil and lemon juice with lemon pepper. It's amazing!).

Choice #3 – Eat breakfast. Breakfast is a great time to establish your daily 3 Rs (reminder, routine, and reward) for eating nutritiously. I personally find if I start the day with the intention of fueling my body with a balance of nutrients, it sets the whole day in order. When our bodies are given the balanced, nutritious fuel it needs, many of our cravings go away. Also, the metabolism kicks in and blood sugar levels don't spike like they do with sugar or high glycemic foods. Sustained energy is the result, along with better weight management! For me, I start my day off with a MyoHealth protein shake and add more nutrients from fruit, fiber, MyoHealth Amino Acids, and Nopalea (for inflammation management). I do this routine five days a week and the other two days, my breakfast consists of eggs, fruit, and one slice of Ezekiel sprouted bread.

Those who eat a balanced fruit/protein and healthy fat breakfast are also less likely to overeat later on. It then becomes much easier to eat several small, evenly spaced portions of food during the day, which is the best way to maintain both blood sugar levels and weight.

Ask Yourself:

Why do I want to eat nutritious food?

____

____

____

____

The problem with most grain cereals is the fact they are highly glycemic, and you have no way of knowing if the grains were grown with pesticides and fertilizers. The combo of high glycemic and foreign invaders with long-term daily intake will sabotage your health.

Quite simply, it's a bad habit that needs to be replaced with a good one!

The CDC (Centers for Disease Control and Prevention) estimates that in the near future, 1 in 3 Americans will have type-2 diabetes ... as a result of our own bad habits. (*diabetes)

I also want to point out one of the biggest health lies ever told was that we need to eat a high carbohydrate and low-fat diet as a general rule for the average consumer. That is pretty much the exact opposite of what our bodies need!

Your brain needs protein and fat! Instead, we starve the brain by going with low fat diets and flood the body with sugars and inflammation by choosing high carbs options. Could those two factors be a contributor in our escalating and almost epidemic rates of dementia and Alzheimer's?

Three world-renowned doctors are speaking out about this very thing, including William Davis, MD, the cardiologist who wrote the *Wheat Belly* books, Brian Perlmutter, MD, the neurologist who wrote the *Grain Brain* books, and Dale Bredesen, MD, who wrote his book on the end of Alzheimer's. If you have not examined some of their research or read their works, you should. It may go against everything you have been told and believed up until this point, but since brain health is important to you, it is worth the read!

Choice #4 – Take nutritional supplements. The more I read and researched to improve my health, the more I became aware of the many nutrients my body was not getting. Most people rarely get sufficient nutrients from the foods they eat. It's nearly impossible, based on the sheer quantity of food needed to get the necessary vitamins and minerals, and it's also highly unlikely that anyone has that variety of food in their house! Therefore, taking supplements is another way to enhance the intake of targeted nutrition and it's quite affordable. You can pay as you go, enjoying a healthy and happy life with less illness and disease ... or you can pay later with doctor and hospital costs as your body, its systems, and its organs weaken over time from the lack of proper nutrition.

Today's aging population has significant chronic lifestyle-related issues that can be traced back to the lack of proper nutrition and the other healthy wellness habits. If they had only started the healthy habits, they would be enjoying the benefits today!

Stress, adrenaline, and lack of sleep had really damaged my body, especially my nervous system. I discovered supplementing my diet with B-12, B-6, and B-9 vitamins helped combat the negative effects of stress, while also restoring my energy and mental clarity. For me, the results were amazing.

Also, research is showing these B vitamins help preserve telomere length, an indicator of your aging process. These are essential factors in the metabolism of the molecules that make up your DNA. Not long ago I took a telomere test and was delighted to know that my chronological age was not a true indicator of how I was really aging. My telomeres had me 24 years younger!

You can buy supplements at countless health food stores and grocery stores, but not all supplements are equal in quality of ingredients or manufacturing standards. You need to find the best source for you. Of course, being the founder of TriVita and having the Senior VP of Supply Chain and Manufacturing of the supplement process report directly to me, I am confident in recommending TriVita's quality high standard supplements. TriVita has an outstanding, quality process with added third-party testing beyond FDA recommended standards to help ensure the ingredients are measured to formula in manufacturing and that what is on the label is in the bottle.

If you want to feel well, eat well.

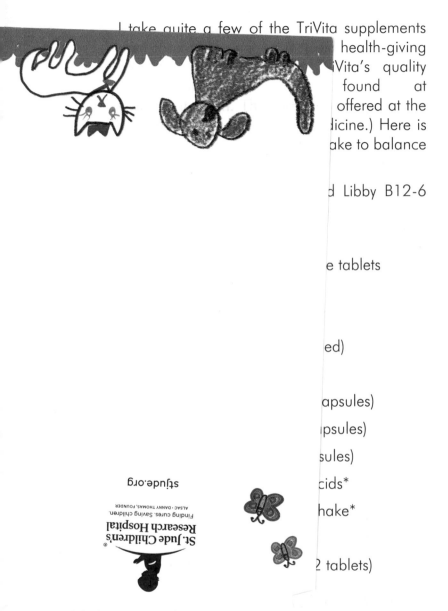

I take quite a few of the TriVita supplements

health-giving

iVita's quality

found at

offered at the

dicine.) Here is

ake to balance

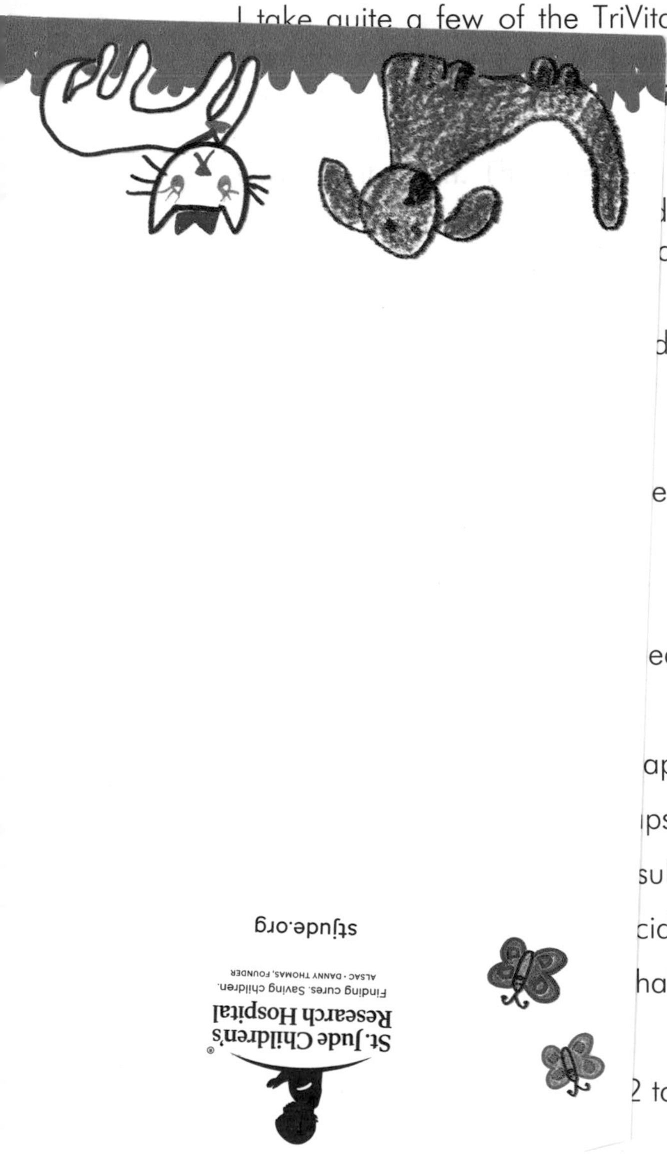

d Libby B12-6

e tablets

ed)

apsules)

psules)

sules)

cids*

hake*

2 tablets)

Make It a Habit

Most people do not make drastic whole-scale dietary changes overnight and stick with them. It's too much change too quickly. That is why I encourage you to establish the habit loop with reminders, routines, and rewards. Take one meal that is routine and set a goal for the nutrient balance you desire. My recommendation is to make it all part of your breakfast! Set up your reminders and repeat often or write down the rewards you are looking for by starting your day with a nutrient blast! You will soon be reaping the rewards of this new habit!

Lasting changes tend to be made one decision at a time, little by little. For me, I made a series of small decisions, and as time passed, I made additional choices that were both practical and creative.

Make Eating Nutritiously a Habit:

When you have a ***reminder*** of what you want, create a ***routine*** of doing what you want, and have a ***reward*** for getting what you want ... you have a habit! You also get what you want!

#1: My reminder is:

____

____

____

#2: My routine is:

____

____

____

#3: My reward is:

____

____

____

Some of those decisions meant trying new cuisines, eating more slowly, and chewing my food more thoroughly. I chose to eat foods that brought me the best nutritional value because I knew that would come back to benefit my body and boost my energy level and give me greater health and a sense of well-being.

You may even want to create a short-term habit of logging what you eat. A lot of people find this helpful because it spells out exactly what they are eating, and that accountability also helps them make wiser food choices. Portion control or eating at specific times can also help as you are creating your food habits.

Whatever habit you are trying to create, use the habit loop of the three Rs by using a reminder, routine, and reward. Life has too many distractions, so habits are the key to get the desired results you want.

The key to the nutrition habit is short and sweet:

> Eat to be well.

The foods you eat and the supplements you take should nourish your body, which in turn should give you the strength and vitality you need to live a happy healthy life with less illness and disease!

That is the habit you want, and it will serve you for a lifetime!

Looking back, it has been more than 20 years since my health crisis. The wellness habit of eating nutritiously has made a significant difference in my health and enjoyment of life since that time. Today, I am enjoying the best health of my life!

Further Reading

*consistent: https://www.webmd.com/food-recipes/features/10-amazing-disease-fighting-foods

*veggies: www.ucsusa.org/11trillionreward

*obesity: https://academic.oup.com/jn/article-abstract/131/3/893S/4687035

*diabetes: https://academic.oup.com/jn/article-abstract/144/4/567S/4571642

Habit #5

Enjoy Activity

The reason for the habit?

– to enjoy life, reduce risk of disease, and fuel a positive attitude

The word "exercise" doesn't usually give people happy thoughts. I have a good friend who just cannot bear the thought of exercising on a consistent basis in the gym or even on a treadmill at home. He is a highly successful individual, but he (like many people) views exercise as boring, repetitive, painful, sweaty, and a chore. They certainly see no fun in that!

But being on the journey toward wellness, we may have to trade in our old way of thinking about physical activity and exercise. We may not be able to get where we want to go – having improved health, greater vitality, higher metabolism, and a stronger immune system – by doing what we've always done.

This two-fold truth most certainly applies:

> First, your well-being requires physical activity (which may include exercising) as that is a natural part of your body's health. Second, this physical activity or exercise does not need to be painful or depressing in order to be

> extremely beneficial to your health and well-being.

Physical activity is a vital part of your overall wellness. There is no substitute or shortcut for physical activity. You need it, your body needs it, and you simply need to find the time so it can become part of your healthy and habitual routine. Just do it! (Thanks Nike!)

Yes, that sounds pretty direct, but I know of no other way to really say it. Physical activity is vitally important. A recent study published in JAMA (one of the most prestigious associations in the nation) tested over 120,000 people and found that exercise (like walking, biking, or running, which increases circulation, respiration, and muscle strength) reduced the chances of dying verses non-exercisers and had no limit in benefits. What is more, the lack of exercise was equal to or worse than cardiovascular disease, diabetes, or smoking.

Did you catch that? What they are saying is this:

> If you are not physically active or do not exercise, the odds of you dying prematurely are greater than if you are a smoker, have diabetes, or heart disease.

Being active and moving is something you do because you desire the health benefits as your reward for your daily routine of physical activity. Perhaps it's not in a local gym. Maybe it's dancing, tennis, walking around your neighborhood or nearest mall with a friend, swimming in the ocean or pool, biking on trails or to and from work, running in the early morning, using a treadmill in your bedroom, or whatever it is you enjoy as a consistent and regular activity that elevates your heart rate and breathing.

Just do something!

Fortunately, my friend has traded in his idea that exercise is a chore and is increasingly physically active, enjoying walking the dog, golfing, and other outdoor activities that keep him moving. As a result, he can reap the health rewards that he wants most.

> The old saying, "No pain, no gain!" is wrong. If one physical activity causes pain, choose another. Find what you enjoy, that helps your body, and then repeat it regularly!

People who stay physically active as long as possible actually live longer lives! It not only helps you live longer, it helps you enjoy the life you have and with less illness and disease.

The secret is to find an activity you enjoy, and then make it a habit. Create the three Rs of the habit loop with reminders, routines, and rewards. Physical activity has the rewards you want. Post your rewards somewhere as your reminder and get in the routine of enjoying physical activity every day!

Someone once said that most any exercise program will work as long as you stick with it.

Find joy and satisfaction in some form of activity. Your body craves it.

You Were Made to Move

Just as the human body was created to breathe, sleep, and heal itself, the human body was also made to move and move often. Regular physical activity offers numerous benefits to your body. Here are 20 benefits that can be yours:

1. Reduced risk of dying from coronary heart disease
2. Reduced risk of having a second heart attack in people who have already suffered one
3. Decreased risk of a stroke
4. Lower high blood pressure
5. Less pain from arthritis
6. Fewer hospitalizations, physician visits, or medications
7. Increased circulation, which speeds oxygen, nutrients, and water to the cells
8. Better functioning lymphatic system, which purges the body of built-up toxins that can lead to disease
9. Bolstered immune system and improved spirit from the release of hormones and enzymes
10. More flexible joints
11. Stronger bones
12. Lower bad cholesterol and triglycerides while raising good cholesterol levels
13. Less risk of developing type 2 diabetes

14. Good muscle tone, vital to looking more youthful
15. More able to handle stress
16. Improved sleep
17. Greater focus and concentration
18. Weight loss
19. More able to keep the weight off
20. Improved physical stamina

Every part of your body, systems, and organs function better when you increase your overall activity level. It just does, and it's tremendous!

You don't need to spend 10 hours a day at the gym to make it happen. Everyone, regardless of age, can benefit from physical activity, even if it's just moderate level activity. It really doesn't take much to get our engines going.

Great Benefits from Walking

I suggest to most people that they make walking their activity habit. If you have been inactive for a while or have serious health concerns, you should see a physician before starting regular physical activity. In most cases, however, a person can begin with a 10-minute walk and not do any harm. Then work up to 30 minutes a day for significant health benefits and cardiovascular disease risk reduction.

Walking is one of the most basic movements. Everyone can do it; a gym membership is not required, and it is highly effective for maintaining and improving our health.

For decades, it has been known that diet and exercise can stop or significantly lessen the slide toward type-2 diabetes.
(*slide)

If done with enough vigor, walking can be an aerobic exercise that conditions your heart and lungs. Even with moderate intensity, walking has both short-term and long-term benefits. Walking is even preferable to jogging or running because walking tends to cause fewer injuries to tendons and joints.

On a side note, if you are walking at dusk or early in the morning, consider wearing reflective tape or clothing to make sure drivers can see you.

Walking is the easiest and best physical activity for most people. Here are some basic walking tips:

- **Invest in a good pair of walking shoes.** You will enjoy walking more and stick with it longer if you have good shoes. Choose shoes with thick, flexible soles that cushion the sole of the foot and absorb shock for the rest of the body.

- **Start slowly.** You should be able to talk while walking and your heart rate should return to normal within 10 minutes after you stop walking.

- **Walk about the same time every day.** Make walking a daily habit that you will "miss" if you don't do it.

- **Increase your distance and speed over time.** Use the first few minutes of a walk to warm up by walking slowly, then gradually increase your speed. Walk slower again at the end of your walk to "cool off."

- **Drink water before and after a vigorous walk.** If you are walking more than 30 minutes, drink water during your walk.

- **Ask someone to walk with you.** It's safer and you will enjoy the exercise more. This can be a good emotional bonding time with a spouse or child.

- **Don't give up.** If you don't reach your goal of time or distance on a given day, don't be

Calculate Your Aerobic Heart Rate

Step #1: 220 - your age = ____ (A)

Step #2: pulse when you wake up = ____ (B)

Step #3: (A) ____ - (B) ____ = ____ (C)

Your aerobic heart rate (optimum fat-burning zone) is 50-75% of (C) + (B) = ____

discouraged. Start again fresh the next morning.

- **Try new routes.** You might try walking through a zoo or park you have not visited in a while.

- **Shake it up.** Once in a while, change your routine, such as going biking, swimming, or running instead, or simply do some extra stretches before you start. A little variety can help you build and maintain a habit.

- **Choose a comfortable time of day.** Nobody enjoys physical activity if it's too hot or too cold.

- **Keep a log of your activity.** Tracking your efforts will motivate you over time. It is one of the best ways to measure your consistent progress.

- **Don't compare yourself to others.** Your goal is your own wellness, not winning a competition. Creating a habit that benefits your life, both now and in the future, is a goal far bigger than any temporary comparison. Be you and be healthy!

When it comes to walking, there is something truly motivating about measuring yourself. In addition to a log to track your activity, I recommend getting a device that counts your footsteps. There are both cheap and more expensive versions, but they all count how many steps you are taking.

People who want to lose weight often find that the closer they get to 10,000 steps a day on a regular basis, the faster the pounds melt away.

> Want to help your heart, protect yourself against diabetes and obesity, lower your blood pressure, improve brain function, and live longer? Exercise more and stay active.
> (*choices)

Set yourself a goal. I suggest aiming for 10,000 steps a day. That's the amount recommended by the President's Council on Physical Fitness and Sports. If you have, for example, 4,000 steps by lunch time, then you know you need to look for ways to boost your steps during the rest of the day. Maybe throw in a walk after dinner. And if your steps are close or over 10,000 in a day, it's gratifying to know you are burning up the calories that day.

Tracking your steps helps you gauge your actual exercise, and that can help motivate you to:

- Park as far from the door of a store entrance as possible.
- Get off of a bus or subway one stop earlier and walk the remaining blocks.
- Take the stairs for several flights instead of the elevator or escalator.

- Get up and walk through your office or outside during coffee and lunch breaks.

Walking is so good for your body. Make it a habit and you will enjoy the benefits that come as a result.

Reconsidering Health Myths

Myths float around in every sphere of life. In the area of physical activity and health, there are plenty of myths. Here are several that need to be replaced with the truth:

Myth #1 – Exercise makes you tired. Moderate activity actually helps reduce fatigue. It energizes your body, gives you strength, and increases your stamina. You may temporarily feel tired as you take steps to create a good physical activity habit, but use that to help you sleep at night!

Myth #2 – Older people should exercise less than younger people. People of all ages need to engage in some form of physical activity. Age is irrelevant. We all benefit from regular physical activity. With older people, exercise

Ask Yourself:

Why do I want to be more active?

____

____

____

____

keeps their bodies healthier, which helps them maintain their independence.

Myth #3 – Exercising with weights makes a person have bulky muscles. Most weight training exercises simply tone the body. That means increased muscle strength without increased muscle size, plus improved bone density. A person at any age can benefit a great deal from activities that use light weights. Though weight loss or maintaining an ideal weight is not the only goal for physical activity, stronger muscles mean a faster metabolism. It has been noted that a pound of muscle burns 50 calories a day, while a pound of fat burns a mere 3 calories per day!

Myth #4 – All physical activities have equal benefits. Some activities have greater benefit to the heart and lungs. These activities include walking, swimming, running, and bicycling, especially with an intensity that causes the heart to pump at an aerobic heart rate level that burns fat. Activities such as stretching help with flexibility and balance but may not push the heart rate up into the aerobic level.

Myth #5 – Unless you are really exercising hard, there are no physical benefits. Even low intensity activities, such as gardening, yard work, housework, and even walking in the grocery store can help lower your risk of heart

> disease, especially if these activities are done daily. Obviously walking briskly has more benefit to the heart and lungs than strolling leisurely, but that leisurely stroll is better than sitting for hours on the couch. In addition, that leisurely stroll might help clear the mind, promote creativity, aid in socialization, and give you a greater appreciation for life as a whole, and those are all good!

When your physical health improves from physical activity, it also benefits you in emotional and psychological ways as well. Countless studies show

Make Being Active a Habit:

When you have a ***reminder*** of what you want, create a ***routine*** of doing what you want, and have a ***reward*** for getting what you want … you have a habit! You also get what you want!

#1: My reminder is:

____

____

____

#2: My routine is:

____

____

____

#3: My reward is:

____

____

____

how increased activity has a beneficial effect on symptoms of depression and anxiety. In addition, regular activity stimulates the growth of new brain cells that enhance memory and learning! Also, regular physical activity helps prevent cognitive decline in older adults.

Take action by getting active. As you would expect, physical exercise boosts your quality of life. One study found that within just two months of getting on an exercise routine, there was a noticeable increase in their quality of life. (*quality)

That's what you want, isn't it?

Make It a Habit

Most health professionals recommend that everyone does at least 30 minutes of physical activity each day. If possible, make it 10 minutes of activity three times a day. Either way, whichever you choose, your body is active and your health is maintained.

> Make it a goal to put in 10,000 steps each day.

I know some people who do 15 minutes of intense exercise each day, and they are very fit. There are many types of equipment that will aid short workouts and deliver outstanding results. I know others who try to spread out their activity so that it lasts all day. They shift up the office space so standing replaces sitting, they walk during coffee breaks, and park at the far end of the parking lot. The end result is a significant increase in life expectancy (*live longer), not to mention being more fit and enjoying life in the moment.

But the only question that matters right now is this one:

> What physical activity are you going to turn into a habit?

A lot of people complain about not having 30 minutes free per day for some form of exercise. Could you find time for several short 10-minute activities of any sort during the day? Maybe a brisk walk, run up the stairs, laps around the office building, or lunch break that requires a 15-minute walk each way. Maybe even a walk, jog, or bike ride around the neighborhood after dinner.

Find something, anything, and stick with it. Then build up your activity slowly over time. Perhaps that means adding more minutes, more steps, more repetitions, or a little heavier weights.

So, have you decided what physical activity you are going to turn into a habit? When your physical activity becomes a habit, it becomes a way of life and contributes greatly to your wellness!

To create your habit, be sure to list your rewards so they are continually enforcing the benefits of your daily routine of physical activity. Then always place those reminders in a visible place so that you don't need to rely on your memory for your daily physical activity habit.

For me, I make the clock my reminder each day. When it is 6:30 AM, it is time to head to the gym! Daily!

Further Reading

*slide: http://care.diabetesjournals.org/content/20/4/537

*choices: http://circ.ahajournals.org/content/94/4/857.full

*quality: https://www.ncbi.nlm.nih.gov/pubmed/10069785

*live longer: https://www.health.harvard.edu/promotions/ harvard-health-publications/cardio-exercise?utm_source=delivra&utm_medium=email&utm_campaign=HB20181027-Cardio&utm_id=1094082&dlv-ga-memberid=56893248&mid=56893248&ml=1094082

Habit #6

Give and Receive Love

The reason for the habit?

> *– to tap into the strongest and greatest motivational force of all*

The journey of wellness is about more than physical health. It also includes emotional, psychological, and spiritual wellness. When they are all combined, you have a strong sense of well-being and are able to pursue and accomplish significant, fulfilling life purposes. In other words:

> Your overall health is measured by how well you manage your body, mind, and soul.

As we shift away from the physical side of wellness, I have found the greatest motivator for changing a mindset and embarking on a wellness journey to be something we often overlook. What is this great motivator? It is this: love.

In the Scriptures, the profound benefits of love are clearly stated, *"And though I bestow all my goods to feed the poor, and though I give my body to be burned but have not love, it profits me nothing. Love suffers long and is kind, love does not envy, love does not parade itself, is not puffed up, does not behave rudely, is not provoked. Love never fails. And now abide faith, hope, love, these three but the greatest of these is love"* (I Cor. 13:3-8a, 13 NKJ).

When I experienced my personal health crisis, I came face to face with what mattered most to me. I found I truly desired two things:

1. To know I was loved
2. To let others know that I loved them

Strangely enough, love was at the root of my choice to change my life. It compelled me to want to get well and it continues to compel me to stay well.

Love is most likely at the core of why people choose the life purposes they do. Love motivates each of us to create or accomplish something beneficial for others. It is love that moves someone beyond "self" to think short-term (necessary daily habits) as well as long-term (life purposes).

> "There is only one happiness in life: to love and to be loved."
> – *George Sand*

All of this is very important, for love gives us purpose. It keeps us going. It motivates us to be whole. As a result, we enjoy life so much more.

The Health Benefits of Love

Love is reflected in our friendships and relationships, and it is here that the benefits of love are so easily seen. Here are just a few of the many benefits that come from loving relationships:

- People in good marriages have a lower risk of cardiovascular disease than those in high-stress relationships. (*married)
- Married people who love each other live longer, have lower cancer rates, and even contract pneumonia less frequently than singles. They are also less likely to suffer from depression, drink heavily, or abuse drugs. What a bonus! (*bonus)
- People in close, loving relationships appear to have significantly higher amounts of immunoglobulin A, an antibody that is the body's first line of defense in fighting disease and infection. (*fighting)
- Hugging may dramatically lower blood pressure and boost blood levels of oxytocin, a relaxing hormone that plays a key role in childbirth labor, breastfeeding, and sexual orgasm. (*hugs)
- Feelings of love and romance release brain chemicals known as neurotransmitters, such as serotonin, dopamine, and norepinephrine. These affect the body in numerous, beneficial ways. For example, people in healthy, happy,

Ask Yourself:

Why do I want to give and receive love?

____

____

____

____

loving relationships are less likely to develop psychological stress disorders, suffer from headaches and back pain, or disengage from physical activity.

But there is more. In fact, there are three distinct, major health benefits directly associated with love. Consider the following:

Benefit #1 – Coherent heart rhythms. Researchers examining heart rhythms and the various factors that create heart rhythm patterns found the heart muscle monitors the blood stream for hormones and translates this hormonal information to the brain. The heart, not the brain, is dictating your body's need for hormones. They also found the autonomic nervous system, which has two branches (one that speeds things up and another that slows things down), is affected by emotions. When you are angry, the two halves of the nervous system get out of sync. One half is trying to speed up the heart and the other half is trying to slow it down, resulting in an erratic rhythm. But when you are in a "loving state," the two halves of the nervous system operate in harmony. This creates a coherent heart rhythm, which helps your body naturally regenerate.

> Loneliness is actually bad for our health.
> (*lonely)

Benefit #2 – Stress hormones defeated. The stress hormone, cortisol, suppresses your immune system. It is released when you are in fight-or-flight situations, including feeling strong anger for only 5 minutes. When cortisol is released, even just for those 5 minutes, it suppresses your body's antibody for up to 6 hours. Lower antibody levels are naturally linked to the increased susceptibility of colds, the flu, nausea, migraines, and even respiratory disease. However, feelings of love and appreciation (even if just for a few minutes) cause antibody levels to rise! The bottom line is that love can boost your immune system, thus counteracting the negative effects of stress. (*destressor) What is more, cortisol can also cause a decrease in DHEA, an anti-aging hormone. Negative emotions (such as anger, hatred, bitterness, and resentment) cause your cells and tissues to age more rapidly. Again, love has the opposite effect. Simply put, if you want to age slower and feel younger, choose love and reject negative emotions.

> Just the memory of a stressful event can cause blood pressure and heart rate to increase.

Benefit #3 – Greater mental health & physical function. Simple acts of caring, helping, and serving generate actual health benefits in return, such as greater mental health and physical function. It literally does your body good to think of others and look for ways to help them, which is showing love at its core. When we have loving relationships, our bodies flourish in countless ways. The list of benefits is long, but the reverse is also true. (*flourish)

Love Is Not Automatic

A lot of people struggle with love, especially in two very important areas. Those who master these two aspects of love are far ahead in the journey of wellness. How would you rate yourself?

The two challenging areas of love that are vital to each one of us and our overall good health include:

Challenge #1 – Loving self. The most difficult lesson for most of us is learning to love ourselves. We are taught from early childhood to give generously and avoid selfishness. This is all good, but not when we feel guilty for doing anything for ourselves; that is a sign that we are out of balance. One very important part of wellness is valuing self. If you don't love you, why take care of yourself, why exercise, and why live a long life? Loving yourself means setting wellness goals that benefit you and creating a habit of giving and receiving love. After all, you are worthy of it! You have every right to give yourself a break, take time to relax, do something that brings personal pleasure, reward yourself in a healthy way, enjoy moments of beauty, and seek to be your best self. You want others to do that for themselves, so you should certainly want that for yourself.

Challenge #2 – Receiving love. The second greatest lesson is learning how to receive love from other people. This applies to those of us who were raised in an environment long on discipline and short on expressions of affection. As a result, we tend to find it difficult to receive gifts or simple expressions of love, such as hugs or tender words. The good news is that we can relearn this and become gracious receivers of love. The key is to stop thinking about ourselves in those moments and think instead, "This is giving the other person pleasure. Don't negate what they are trying to do." If you dismiss someone's compliment, applause, or expressions of love toward you, you are rejecting their gift and calling them dishonest. Never devalue acts of love from someone. After all, you wouldn't want them to devalue your expressions of appreciation, approval, or love toward them, would you?

"To love someone is to see a miracle invisible to others." – *Francois Mauriac*

It seems strange to tell people that they need to love themselves and receive love from other people. It's almost like reminding people to eat food or sleep, because you would think that loving yourself and

Make Giving & Receiving Love a Habit:

When you have a ***reminder*** of what you want, create a ***routine*** of doing what you want, and have a ***reward*** for getting what you want ... you have a habit! You also get what you want!

#1: My reminder is:

____

____

____

#2: My routine is:

____

____

____

#3: My reward is:

____

____

____

receiving love would be natural ... but it's not! That is the scary part.

Our bodies function so much better when we give ourselves what we truly need, and love is an unquestionably important ingredient in our overall health.

For me, learning to receive love was quite difficult. Expressions of love, such as hugs or words of affirmation, were not part of my family upbringing. We were very cause oriented and performance driven, but love was soft and uncomfortable. The best advice I can give to those who were raised like me is to simply say "thank you" to anyone expressing to you their care, appreciation, kindness, or even praise.

Make It a Habit

How do you give love? How do you show love? How do you make giving and receiving love a practical part of your daily routine?

There are countless ways to do so, but one of the simplest and most practical expressions of love that I have found is sending a note or card.

My wife and I love the seasons and times of the year when we can express our love to each other in a card. We both go to great effort looking for the special card that says just the right things for where we are in life. These cards always demonstrate the love and affection we have for each other, wrapped in our special message (I have saved 50 years of cards from her with all her special love notes!).

> Love helps your body heal. (*heal)

You might:

- Choose a blank card and write a message in it
- Send a touching quote or find a card with that special message of love you want to convey
- List at least one quality, act of kindness, or character trait that you admire or respect in the person

It's an incredibly fun exercise. I challenge you to pause right now and jot down a quick list of people who need to hear you say, "I love you." It can also be an expression of "I admire you" or "I respect you."

Later, take the time to send a little note to each of the people on your list over the course of the next 6 months. You can do that. It's easy.

> "The best and most beautiful things in this world cannot be seen or even heard, they must be felt with the heart." – *Helen Keller*

Keep loving on yourself and keep loving on others. The act of giving and receiving love is not only enjoyable, it is necessary for your health.

One of the most powerful demonstrations of the power of the words "I love you" was at the ceremonial burial services of President George H.W. Bush. When his son, President George W. Bush, concluded his remarks honoring his passing father, he said the last words he spoke to his father were, "Dad, I love you," to which his father had replied, "Son, I love you." George W. Bush could not contain his stiff upper lip and broke into crying with overwhelming love!

To best create the habit of giving love, you will need to focus on the routines of your life and then set reminders until these form the habit of giving and receiving love. The rewards to you, your wellness, and to those receiving your love will be amazing!

The calendar of seasons is both a reminder and routine to establish giving cards and notes of love and appreciation. Grandchildren are also the perfect way of getting comfortable in verbalizing your words of love and admiration. It is your opportunity to create the habit of giving love, and getting love returned, with so many wellness benefits.

You are meant to enjoy the habit of giving and receiving love!

Further Reading

*married: https://www.reuters.com/article/us-health-marriage /marriage-tied-to-lower-risk-of-fatal-heart-attacks-and-strokes-idUSKBN1JE2XG

*bonus: https://www.webmd.com/sex-relationships/features/ health-benefits#1

*fighting: https://www.hyperbiotics.com/blogs/recent-articles/ how-love-improves-your-health-and-impacts-your-life

*hugs: https://www.dailymail.co.uk/health/article-2266373 /Hugging-lower-blood-pressure-boost-memory.html

*lonely: http://time.com/5136409/health-benefits-love/

*destressor: https://www.huffpost.com/entry/love-health-benefits_b_3131370

*flourish: https://www.ncbi.nlm.nih.gov/pmc/articles/PMC 3537144/

*heal: https://www.ncbi.nlm.nih.gov/pubmed/15990734

Habit #7

Be Forgiving

The reason for the habit?

– to set yourself emotionally free to pursue your highest purposes

Strange as it may sound, I think everyone past their first birthday has felt some emotional pain. That's just the world we live in. Of course, the hurt comes in a variety of forms. Maybe it was rejection from a group on the playground, insults or criticism, teasing, bullying, the loss of a friendship, unjustified punishment, or even abuse.

As we mature in life, we may experience loss in the form of a job termination, divorce, or abusive relationships. Whatever or whoever the cause, and regardless of the severity of the actual pain, these emotional wounds tend to cut deep and remain unhealed.

Then, when we hang on to hurt, either consciously or subconsciously, heartache develops that can seethe just beneath the surface of other emotions. That wound can give rise to outbursts of anger, feelings of revenge or deep shame, and guilt. Here is the challenge:

> Painful emotions can become toxic, and that cannot lead to a full and healthy life. In fact,

> many people suffer serious health issues that are anchored in an unforgiven incident or events in their lives.

The bad news is that most of us don't know we have been holding on to toxic emotions for years, even decades. The longer we hold on to negative emotions, the less likely we are to wish for change. The anger, hate, revenge, or shame is "who we are," even though it's not. We have all heard the phrase, "That's just who I am."

What would it be like to be free? Do we even want to be free of the emotional pain? It feels so right when we have been so wronged!

I have found that when we dig down to the core issue behind the reluctance to let go of the pain, there is a thread of logic that reasons:

> "If I let go, doesn't that let the other person get away with what they have done to me?"

But trying to hold someone accountable or even captive for their past actions toward you seldom brings real justice, nor does it do anything to lessen the pain. And sadly, this creates a chemical imbalance in every cell in your body as you try to function optimally, though your body cannot.

A report from Johns Hopkins Medicine on forgiveness said that unforgiveness and the emotions that accompany it can increase the risk of heart disease, blood pressure and stroke, diabetes, depression, weight gain, and other health risks. No thanks!

More than likely, unforgiveness holds you in bondage while the other person moves on with life. And that makes it twice as bad, because they hurt you the first time, and then they walk away, perhaps without any direct consequences for their actions, and you are the one still hurting! This also can become habit forming, as each time the person or incident is thought of, the brain sends out an emotional chemical release through the body, and your cells feel that chemical stimulant and respond, making you further dependent on the emotional trigger of hurt to feel anger or resentment.

How then can we break free? How can we bring healing to our very real emotional pain? The answer is this:

Choose to forgive so that you can be free.

Just like love, giving and receiving forgiveness is essential to your wellness. Forgiveness is one of the most powerful forms of healing! It is our way to God in restoring relationship, no matter to what degree our sinfulness!

Genuine Forgiveness

What is forgiveness? I have seen some crazy definitions and examples of forgiveness. Some of them

Ask Yourself:

Why do I want to forgive?

____

____

____

____

are so twisted and convoluted that it's no wonder people struggle to forgive.

Here is the deal. Be honest with yourself! Do you want the rewards of forgiveness? No matter how difficult it might be, the rewards are there for you. This is not a logical experience, but rather an act of supernatural power released when you forgive.

When it comes to forgiveness, you must first answer this question:

> **Question #1 – Do I want to be free?** Forgiveness is letting go. It is releasing negative hurt and heartaches, releasing the emotions associated with painful experiences, and releasing the person who hurt you from the prison of your heart.

In letting go and releasing the other person, you are setting yourself free from the grip of unforgiveness.

It is vitally important in your quest for freedom to understand clearly what forgiveness is NOT:

- **Forgiveness is NOT ...** saying the negative experience never happened, that it was not painful, or that it was wrong for you to feel pain. Forgiveness is not denial.
- **Forgiveness is NOT ...** saying that everything is "okay." Forgiveness is not glossing over a wrong and saying that it does not matter.
- **Forgiveness is NOT ...** saying that all claims to justice need to be laid aside. Wrongs should be righted or compensated, and negative situations and relationships should be healed

> and reconciled. Justice should prevail. In some cases, perpetrators or abusers need to be arrested, charged, and convicted in a court of law. Compensation for losses and retribution may need to take place. At the least, apologies should be spoken. However, there is just one catch. You are not the person who can usually make things right. It takes two people to reconcile a relationship, and it takes a higher authority to administer justice. You do not have control or authority over the person who hurt you.

Then comes another question:

> **Question #2 – How do I let go?** Forgiveness means letting go, but how do you do that? It begins by choosing not to carry those negative and toxic emotions around in your heart any longer. It means you choosing to release those long-held emotions, choosing to release the memory of that situation, and choosing to release the person who hurt you from the dungeon of your heart.

Yes, it requires a lot of choosing, but that is what it takes. You must choose it. Nobody else can choose it for you. I have witnessed people go through unimaginable pain, torment, and abuse, but by choosing to walk out their forgiveness, they are as free as a bird today. They are light, happy, joyful, and overflowing with exuberant life! They are free, and it's amazing to see them now, knowing what they experienced in the past.

As for the person who did the wrong? More than likely, their life is in shambles. Those who cause pain are seldom whole, healthy, vibrant people. But I have seen sometimes where those who have done wrong and harm seem to live above their abusive behavior.

It truly doesn't matter. The power of forgiveness is not based on retribution. Forgiveness brings you freedom, regardless of the other person.

You and I can be healed and restored. Forgiveness sets us free!

Why Is Forgiveness So Important?

Walking in forgiveness by choosing to forgive is important on many levels. Perhaps you can answer these questions:

- If you hold on to what is negative, can you really receive what is positive and helpful into your life?
- If you contemplate revenge, can you simultaneously think creative, productive, wholesome, enriching, and honorable thoughts?
- If you harbor hatred, can you feel love?
- If you are full of anger, can you be an instrument of peace at the same time?
- If you hold on to old, painful memories, can you create new, beautiful memories?
- If you cling to broken relationships, can you establish healthy relationships?

Without question, to genuinely improve our well-being and happiness, not to mention our health, we must forgive … and that enables us to let go of the pain.

I have found there to be several truths about forgiveness that always apply, without exception:

1. No matter how healthy all of your other habits are, unless you forgive, you will never feel your best physically, emotionally, or spiritually.
2. Letting go of negative feelings allows peace and optimism to flow into you in a new and powerful way.
3. Not all forgiveness happens instantly, but the beginning of forgiveness happens at the moment you choose to forgive.

Forgiveness is an act of the will. It is the first step in the right direction. You may not arrive at perfect peace and joy instantly, but you can rest assured that you are going in the right direction and that peace and joy will come as you continue to walk out forgiveness.

Anger and hostility are actually linked to heart disease.
(*heart)

Years ago, I was deeply hurt by two people at my business. The loss was significant on many levels, especially at the financial level. I struggled with forgiveness, but I knew that in order to be better, I needed to make a conscious choice to not be bitter. Though I wasn't sure how to release the bitterness, I did recognize I could choose to either be bitter or better. If you have struggled in your life with hurt and pain, you can also make the choice between being bitter and better, and that alone can start the healing process!

One day it came to me. I had previously planted two small palm trees by the tennis court at my home and they had gotten sick. I named those two palm trees the names of the individuals who caused me so much pain in my business, and then did everything I could to help the trees recover. In addition, every time I went to play tennis, I walked by those trees and said, "I bless you."

Build Up Your Emotional Immunity:

When we tell someone, "I forgive you," we are also saying, "There is no longer an issue between us." You are free of any hold they had on you. You have a new confidence and freedom to speak and act because you are no longer concerned about what they think, say, or do.

You may even find you don't mind being around that person as much as you did. This does not mean you should automatically open yourself up to them with total trust. Hurting people hurt people, so unless they have changed, they will do it again.

By forgiving, you can hold your head high and refuse to cower or shrink in the presence of those who hurt you. When you let go of people and your pain, you free yourself from internalizing their criticism or hatred. You have a higher degree of emotional immunity!

An amazing thing happened ... my anger and bitterness melted away. I was able to focus on rebuilding my business and my life rather than ruminating on my anger, disappointment, and hurt. I was free! My health and emotions were strengthened.

My business recovered and grew again, and those two trees did the same and are standing tall to this day.

Can You Forgive Yourself?

Do you find it difficult to forgive yourself? I think most people do. They might be able to forgive someone else, but when it comes to forgiving themselves, that is often where they draw the line.

But just like learning to love yourself (as mentioned in the last chapter) is important, so is learning to forgive yourself. But...

- Maybe the past mistakes and failures are just "too big" to forgive
- Maybe the guilt acts as a motivator
- Maybe you don't think you are worthy of forgiveness

In the end, choosing not to forgive yourself leaves you in a miserable condition, and that often leads to very poor health habits, addictive behaviors, and a whole lot of stress, all of which invite illness and disease.

As for guilt, I am convinced that much of the guilt people feel toward themselves is false guilt. This false guilt is based on unreasonably high standards of performance. Of course, nobody can ever achieve perfection, but the pursuit of perfection and the failure to attain it can cause false guilt.

Another common cause for false guilt occurs when we have been hurt in childhood and then feel guilty later for things we could not then control. This often occurs with child molestation, a crime that happens far more than we want to recognize as a society.

> Want to boost your self-esteem? Choose to forgive!
> (*self-esteem)

Many people today suffer guilty feelings, thinking that, somehow, they as a child were responsible for what happened. That is not the case! I encourage anyone who may have had this happen to them to seek professional counseling to find forgiveness and peace with themselves.

It's really just taking responsibility for negative behaviors that we did not cause yet, for some reason, think we started. How unfortunate is that?

As for guilt, it is important that you know:

> Guilt is specific, and it is based on something you did. Take responsibility for it and move on. Throw false guilt aside. It is not yours to worry about. Throw it out, let it go, and move on!

If you find it necessary to take out the trash of any false guilt, you will find it necessary to throw out old memories associated with rejection, hurt, and failure as well.

Many years ago, I did something that brought me great freedom. I had previously come to see some of my own behaviors that may have hurt people, though not intentionally. I took responsibility for any potential hurt I may have caused someone and wrote letters to the people who were involved and asked for their forgiveness.

I also wrote letters to those who had hurt me, telling them I was forgiving them for the hurt I had experienced and explaining that I was setting the memory of the hurt free from my mind and heart and asked them to do the same.

These letters were sometimes many pages long. It took me quite a while to write all the letters. Writing a detailed letter was a tangible way of scraping out of my heart the negative emotions and guilt that had become encrusted there.

When I was done, I mailed some, but threw, shredded, or burned most of them. Why not mail all of them? In nearly every situation, the person involved would not have remembered the incident or did not think there was an issue between us.

> Make it a practice to let go of bad memories.

In several cases, the person was dead. I mailed a few that were relevant and necessary. But whether I mailed them or not, the point for me was that I needed to forgive and let go, and to forgive myself for any pain I had caused. I needed to move on.

Of course, in some situations, mailing a letter to someone might not be appropriate. For me, it was an internal exercise that set me free, brought me peace, and improved my health. It was life changing on my wellness journey.

When it comes to forgiveness and forgiving myself, I have often pondered these words:

> Another person may not need to know that you forgive them or that you want to be forgiven by them. YOU are the one who needs to know that you have forgiven and released the issue so that it's no longer an issue. Forgiveness is primarily for YOUR sake.

There is freedom in forgiveness!

How to Get the Peace You Desire

Forgiveness is the foundation for living with an inner sense of peaceful well-being. In other words, if you want peace, you must learn to forgive and continue to live in a place of forgiveness. Without forgiveness, there cannot be true peace.

And as you know, it is also good for your health. Forgiveness can bring a significant decrease in symptoms such as chest pain, back pain, headaches, sleep problems, nausea, and loss of appetite.

There are a lot of physical "ailments" that are caused in part by troubled heart and mind.

To achieve this much needed peace, which comes from working through forgiveness, people have come up with numerous techniques to achieve that goal. Here is one that I have found to be very effective:

Step #1 – Tell your grievance story. Say it once as fully as possible. Write it down if necessary.

Step #2 – Never repeat it. Once you have told your grievance story, refuse to tell it again. Rehearsing a grievance or grudge only engrains it in your emotions. Each retelling of the story raises your blood pressure and pumps adrenaline into your system.

Step #3 – Replace the old story. Now that the old grievance story is gone, you need to create a new story about what you desire for your life. Talk about the attributes you want to have in your relationships with other people, including the person who hurt you. At times, you may want to have distance or separation in a relationship, and that is fine. Recognize that for distance or separation to be completely satisfactory, you must want the other person to have some degree of peace and joy in their life, as you have peace and joy in yours.

Step #4 – Move on to something else. If anger or unrest surfaces when faced with the old memories, do something else with your time. Maybe start a practical project that gets you busy and is completely separate from the feelings and thoughts that you are associated with your situation. Find a way to move on mentally and physically.

This process is simple, and it works. I've suggested a few steps, but you may know of another technique that you prefer.

Do whatever it takes for you to walk out forgiveness so you can have the peace you want, need, and deserve.

More Health Benefits of Forgiveness

What happens when you choose to forgive? There is breakthrough, peace, restored hope, joy, boldness, creativity, and so much more.

These emotional and psychological benefits are not only great, they are also sometimes immediate. But there is more. Here are five common physical benefits that are repeatedly associated with forgiveness:

Benefit #1 – Reduced stress. When we are stressed, our muscles tense, blood pressure rises, and sweating increases. All three of these symptoms are significantly reduced or even reversed as we forgive.

Benefit #2 – Reduced pain. When we trade our anger and bitterness for compassion and forgiveness, we feel less pain. Anxiety associated with pain also decreases.

Benefit #3 – Better heart health. There is a strong link between forgiveness and improvements in our blood pressure and heart rate. When we forgive, we decrease the workload on our heart muscle.

Benefit #4 – Improved brain function and memory. Replacing our old, negative memories with happier memories means we have more brain power available to create, problem solve, and make good decisions, all of which contribute to a greater quality of life.

Benefit #5 – Stronger immune function. After we choose to forgive, unhealthy hormones and chemicals stop being released into our bloodstream, which naturally has a positive effect on our good hormones and neurotransmitters.

Interestingly, these benefits associated with forgiveness seem to increase with age. This makes sense if you think about it because the older we get, the more issues, baggage, negativity, hurt, and pain that can accumulate. When we let go and choose to forgive, we drop the emotional, mental, and psychological weight of past hurt, which translates directly into the physical realm. Forgiveness lightens our burdens. (*load)

As you know, time alone does not heal, nor does it bring about forgiveness. Instead, it is through forgiveness that we find the healing we need. It is a process, something we can learn how to do. (*learning) Even if the issue is decades old, forgiveness still works beautifully!

One of the greatest prayers of forgiveness recorded in history was when Jesus prayed while hanging on the cross for crimes he did not commit, and said, *"Father, forgive them for they do not know what they do."* (Luke 23:34 NKJ).

It is a profound example of the power of forgiveness and the model of simply taking the first step toward releasing forgiveness in your life. Forgiving is in the act of speaking forgiveness, not in the act of forgetting.

Make It a Habit

Once you have chosen to forgive yourself or another person by releasing old, hurtful memories, it is important that you keep choosing to forgive. Feel free to say aloud, "I forgave that person. I forgive and let it go right now."

Feel free to write letters, asking and giving forgiveness. Some letters you will need to mail, others you'll need to throw away. Do it to get free.

Repeating this as often as you need to will help cement the forgiveness into your heart and mind.

This is all part of your commitment to ongoing forgiveness. Refuse to allow negative and toxic emotions to entrap you again. They are bad for your health and wellness, so keep up a guard so they don't get in.

As you are walking through forgiveness, it is important that you give yourself permission to love again, to trust again, and to reach

Make Forgiveness a Habit:

When you have a ***reminder*** of what you want, create a ***routine*** of doing what you want, and have a ***reward*** for getting what you want ... you have a habit! You also get what you want!

#1: My reminder is:

____

____

____

#2: My routine is:

____

____

____

#3: My reward is:

____

____

____

out again to help other people. Resist the urge to shrink back from doing the right things out of fear of pain and hurt. Take the risk.

The more you practice forgiveness, the easier it will be to risk loving and giving again because you know that if people hurt you, you can forgive and walk freely and confidently with hope toward your own future. Nobody can hold you down!

Lastly, remember that forgiveness is a process, not just a moment. Enjoy the journey toward a life in which you live in complete forgiveness of others and yourself.

If you learn and practice the 3 Rs habit loop of forgiveness in small ways, you will be better prepared to forgive the unfortunate, big things that happen in life.

What are the routine things in life that would give you the opportunity to forgive and be forgiven? Identify the reminders and rewards to make forgiving a habit, which will directly promote health and well-being in your life.

Find your two palm trees, like I did, to remind you to not only forgive but to bless those who have hurt you. When you do, you release God's blessings into your life!

Further Reading

*heart: https://www.ncbi.nlm.nih.gov/pubmed/19281923

*self-esteem: https://www.mayoclinic.org/healthy-lifestyle/adult-health/in-depth/forgiveness/art-20047692?p=1

*load: https://journals.sagepub.com/doi/abs/10.1177/1948550614564222

*learning: https://www.hopkinsmedicine.org/health/healthy_aging/healthy_connections/forgiveness-your-health-depends-on-it

Habit #8

Practice Gratitude

The reason for the habit?

– to maintain a thankful attitude for the now and in anticipation of the future

Gratitude is expressed through thankfulness, and the people who are the most thankful always seem to have a magnetic, friendly, positive attitude. In addition, they are the people we want to be around, are they not?

Before my health crisis, I was grateful for the many things I had accomplished, acquired, and experienced. But gratitude was not a strong emotion for me, and I would certainly say I was not intentional about expressing gratitude through thankfulness.

Like most people, it's easy to get caught up in the hustle and bustle of life and its demands, and little by little we forget to appreciate the blessings all around us. When we are under stress, with demands on our time and energy, our focus shifts to the negatives, the worries, the frustrations, and our expectations of people and of our owns efforts!

As a direct result, we can easily lose sight of what we appreciate the most in life and instead focus on what we expect in life.

Embracing gratitude opens the door to a new way of looking at life. It is an invitation to celebrate the joy and beauty life offers in so many ways.

Being grateful does not mean you need to repay anyone for anything. Gratitude is not a tit-for-tat requirement. Real gratitude is a sincere appreciation for something, anything, whether you can repay it or not. Love given does not require repayment. A beautiful sunrise or sunset does not suspend itself waiting for your applause or appreciation. The sun comes up and goes down, and every farmer is grateful for it, yet nothing is owed in return.

Gratitude is an attitude, not rent or interest that must be repaid. It is free, but it benefits you greatly.

Gratitude Always Fits

We are all passionate creatures, filled with feelings, opinions, and thoughts about everything around us. These feelings, opinions, and thoughts are a big part of who we are and how we experience life. They give us feedback, which helps us act with better direction and purpose in our lives. As a result, we thrive on feeling good and endlessly look for ways to avoid pain.

What, then, is gratitude? Does it make you feel good or does it bring pain (discomfort, repayment, indebtedness)? Without question, gratitude is a feel-good experience! There is no pain in it whatsoever.

But it's not all about fun and pleasure. Don't we often learn the most during difficult, trying times? You bet! And that is something we can, and should, all be grateful for! And can you be grateful for things you didn't experience, such as not living during the Dark Ages, not having to stand in line for hours for food, or not losing family members to diseases that have been eradicated so many years ago?

Being grateful for all that we have, even for the tough times, creates such a positive outlook on life. That is an incredible reward in and of itself.

But gratitude was a habit I needed to choose to develop. It did not come naturally to me. I was, like a lot of people, in achievement mode. I didn't inherit any money or receive any unexpected windfalls, so I knew from an early age that any degree of success in life would be the result of my own hard work, ingenuity, and skill. I always believed in the purpose of God and His blessings, but I also believed in the effort of man. If I wanted anything, I was going to have to go after it to get it.

Balance is vital if we are trying to enjoy life.

Up to the age of 50, I spent my years setting, pursuing, and reaching goals. Some goals were personal, some were business, some involved family, and some concerned church and community. What I had never considered before, but now realize, is that:

> Passionate pursuit must be balanced by deep gratitude.

When I started on the journey of wellness, I recognized the obvious fact that I needed to rethink and reshape my entire life. Was my overly competitive drive really getting me what I wanted?

The short answer: No!

For years I had ignored the glaring fact that my intense striving to achieve goals brought me pain (physical and relational) and weakness (emotional and relational) rather than joy, favor, or blessing. It was very hard for me to admit that in all my winning, I was still coming out ahead. I was so far out of balance that there was no way to "tweak it" or "refine my focus." It was broken, and it needed to be fixed!

I ignored it. But when faced with pre-mature death, I had no choice but to address the reality I lived in. With so much to fix, where could I begin? I started by telling myself regularly:

> I'm grateful to be alive, grateful to have a chance to redo some things, grateful for a loving family to help me through this, and grateful I can still think and make changes.

Before long, I found myself grateful for simple things, such as a long night of sleep, renewed energy, less physical pain, and any sign of returning strength. We live in Arizona where the sunsets are spectacular, and they have become my reminder for the habit of gratitude and to experience the reward of good feelings when I express my gratitude.

The Mindset for Health

Wellness is not a destination but a journey. This mindset allows each one of us to experience a fuller and richer life. Making the habits of wellness a part of our daily journey contributes directly to a happier and healthier life with less sickness and disease.

The journey to wellness required a whole new mindset for me. I could not do what I had always done and expect better results. That would never happen.

I discovered wellness is not a goal to be achieved but a life of choices to be lived. I could not say "Okay, I did it, and now I'm done." Wellness is truly a journey, a lifelong journey that you get to enjoy along the way. There is no wellness trophy you can win, nor is it something you can tick off your checklist.

> If gratitude improves our self-image and makes us more attractive, why aren't we always overflowing with gratitude?
> (*attractive)

And because wellness is a journey, we have to change our mindset to fit this new reality.

This new mindset includes practicing the habit of gratitude, and to do that we must be cognizant of the 3 Rs in the habit loop (reminder, routine, and reward). This changes our behavior from trying to remember to be grateful to actually doing it.

Much research has already established the fact that our mind wants to create a habit response rather than constantly having to rationalize a conscious action. Your mind prefers that you act, behave, decide, and think based on your habits. This applies all the time, whether your behavior is good or bad. Habits require little thinking, which is what the mind prefers.

Why do some children throw temper tantrums or compulsively beg? Because their mind has decided it works in most cases, so whenever they don't get what they want, their habit response kicks in. Parents frequently fall into that trap and that reinforces the habitual behavior.

Research in the neurobiochemistry of thought explains that as we connect a thought-feeling with a certain kind of event, or thoughts and feelings with each other, we strengthen the neurological web of reaction. In short, it becomes a mental habit.

When we repeatedly relive the same angry emotions attached to an event or person, we are literally strengthening the brain to automatically think and feel that same anger. Naturally, our emotional anger becomes physically bigger and stronger as it is tied to those related events and feelings. With anger comes a hormonal response, which create feelings throughout the body and its cells. Each repetition makes the negative response all the more habitual.

This type of negative habit loop has the event as the reminder, which triggers the routine of anger, and the body thinks the rush of emotions are its reward. After all, it feels natural, and the mind has chosen to justify the habit.

This may also help explain why it is so difficult to change emotional habits, even when we truly desire to change them.

Not long ago, I was in an interview and the moderator asked me if he could create good health habits without giving up bad habits, such as starting his day with just coffee and doughnuts. I explained how wellness is not about giving up bad habits but about creating new, good habits that, over time, will take over and give you what you want. The bad habits will naturally fall away.

If we apply this to the habitual anger explained above, how would that look? Let's say you want to do away with the anger response and replace it with the mindset of gratitude and its good feelings. You can create the mindset of experiencing the rewards of gratitude. Maybe the rising sun is your reminder to begin your routine of being thankful for life, beauty, health, strength, the benefits of the sun, food, and so much more. The rising sun is a perfect start to a habit of gratitude. Eventually, the gratitude will start to overlap and eventually drown out the anger habit. I don't think anything can stand up to a habit of gratitude!

Today, I enjoy life far more than I did before. While I am admittedly still on the journey of wellness, I still maintain my focus on the other aspects of life (business, growth, networking, leaving a legacy, helping others, etc.) that I value, but I have learned to do life with balance.

What gave me the greatest push toward balance was being thankful. I was thankful for the "little things," such as time with my grandkids, connecting with

Ask Yourself:

Why do I want to learn to be grateful?

____

____

____

____

someone, going for a walk with my wife, or taking a moment to help someone with their own concerns. Those things were all time well spent! I never would have thought so before my health scare, but after facing premature death, I am truly thankful that I can be here and participate in life.

Gratitude often requires an adjustment in priorities.

It is a journey, and when we are grateful to be on it, we have much more joy and balance because of it.

Develop an Attitude of Gratitude

If you are like me, an attitude of gratitude is not going to suddenly appear and fall into your lap by magic. It's going to take some work. It will take conscious effort, but most of all, it will require you to create the habit of gratefulness.

You can learn to experience the good feelings of gratitude daily by setting up reminders in your daily routines. In the beginning, those reminders need to be your clue to offer an expression or thought of gratitude. Make it a natural habit, and then enjoy the amazing rewards!

Learning to express gratitude is pretty simple. It means sincerely saying such things as:

- "Thank you."
- "I appreciate you and what you teach me through your life."

- "I'm grateful to you for the example you are and the work you do."

Who is worthy of your gratitude? Anyone who contributes to your life in a positive way is worthy, and that includes everyone who gives you their time, talent, or skills. When you stop and think about it, that's a lot of people!

You must take action on your gratefulness to start the process of turning it into a habit. These 3 steps can help:

> **Step #1** – Take a moment and ask yourself: "What am I most grateful for today?"
>
> **Step #2** – Then, pull out a notebook and make a list of the top 25 things for which you are most grateful. If people are on list, have you thanked that person for being in your life, loving you, and giving to you? Have you thanked the person lately? Ever? Today?
>
> **Step #3** – Show your appreciation practically with a note, letter, email, gift, phone call, or a quick face-to-face chat.

The more you focus on what you are grateful for, the more you will shift your focus from what you do NOT have to what you DO have. This shift in perspective can be as dramatic as a sudden earthquake! And the effect is usually profound.

It is important to recognize that at a deeper level, gratitude is more than a spoken word or note of thanks. It is a perspective, an attitude, that is evident by what you say, think, and do.

An attitude of gratitude is developed over time as you place value on what truly matters.

Benefits of Gratitude

I have found, and no doubt you have as well, that when we focus on what we don't have, we tend to get frustrated, anxious, worried, and all around grumpy. Hope seems to fade, and that often leads to discouragement, which is only a few steps away from depression and despair.

This is a long downhill slope, and it began all the way back at discontentment, comparison, and a lack of gratitude. How sad is that?

However, when we focus on the good things we DO have in life, it is hard not to have a positive, uplifting attitude as a direct result. We are even more likely to help other people in need. (*others) This attitude often leads to a positive expectancy, almost an increased level of alertness, of what is to come. Life is good, and it's only going to get better!

> When gratitude is the soil, all relationships can be improved.

Gratitude directly gives way to enthusiasm for life, which naturally brings with it determination, optimism, and energy. And instead of hopelessness, there is a deep sense of joy.

Here are several direct benefits of having an attitude of gratitude:

1. More satisfaction
2. Increased sense of purpose
3. Fulfillment
4. Positive thoughts
5. Hope
6. Greater faith
7. Unstoppable optimism
8. Happiness
9. Better mood
10. Peace

I read about a psychologist, Robert Emmons, who spent decades studying what makes people happy. He concluded:

> "When people consciously practice grateful living, their happiness will go up, and their ability to withstand negative events will improve."

Choose to be grateful.

Here are even more benefits to consider:

11. Gratitude causes relationships to improve because it gives you more empathy and makes you more generous.
12. Grateful people have wider and stronger social networks.

13. Grateful people feel more responsibility for others.

14. Grateful people are less envious.

But there is more! There are physical health benefits of gratitude as well. Grateful people often:

15. Exercise more regularly.

16. Report fewer physical symptoms of illness.

17. Exhibit more energy.

18. Sleep longer and better.

19. Feel better about their lives as a whole.

20. Possess more optimism about the future.

These are amazing benefits. If that is not enough, did you know that optimistic people routinely have higher numbers of blood cells that protect the immune system, so they fare better during surgery and respond to treatment quicker than pessimists?

Gratitude Looks Forward:

Expressing gratitude includes expressing gratitude for things that have not yet happened but believe will become real in the future. When you give thanks in advance for things that have not occurred, your mind and heart have positive expectancy. When you live that way, it creates an atmosphere of gratitude where creativity thrives, and that produces the very things you desire most!

And the actual physical effects of thankfulness last in the body and brain for months afterward – all from being grateful! (*lasting) I never knew what I was missing!

Amazingly, we can choose to be grateful even if we don't feel very thankful. Why would we do that? Because emotions with feelings follow thoughts! When we choose to concentrate on the blessings in life, we see more and more good things. Feeling thankful is the direct result.

Abraham Lincoln knew this when he said:

> "Most folks are as happy as they make up their minds to be."

When we lead with thankfulness, our heart and head will follow. Practice takes work, but when it's a habit, it truly becomes part of us.

Make It a Habit

Perhaps the simplest way to make gratitude a habit is to keep a gratitude journal. Every day, or at least once a week, write down the things for which you are grateful. From time to time, take a few extra minutes to write down why you are grateful for these things in your life.

> If you keep a gratitude journal, you can expect greater health, better sleep, lower blood pressure, more energy, and MUCH more!
> (*journal)

I know a family that gathers around every few months and reads the previous list before writing down their new gratitude items. It's a great way of remembering the past and tracking the present.

Here are a few suggestions to get your list of thankfulness flowing:

- Who are you grateful for, both past and present?
- Which physical talents and abilities are you thankful for?
- What experiences are you grateful for, both past and present?
- What decisions or choices have you made that are benefitting you now?
- What opportunities are you grateful for?
- Have unexpected and enjoyable things happened to you recently?
- How is your physical, emotional, and spiritual health?
- What is it about nature that makes you say, "Wow"?

I saw a great anonymous quote that read:

> "If you can't be thankful for what you receive, be thankful for what you escape."

How true is that?

You may want to list in your journal the things you don't have to experience, such as problems that are not yours, and that can help you see the many blessings that are yours. Along those lines, inspirational speaker and author Denis Waitley put it this way:

> "I had the blues because I had no shoes until upon the street, I met a man who had no feet."

Makes you think, doesn't it?

As you journal the many reasons you have to be thankful, reflect once in a while on your longstanding relationship with a spouse, child, or friend. This also counts in your relationship with God. Contemplate all the many blessings that come from God, your family, and your friends. You will quickly find yourself welling up with gratitude.

Make Gratitude a Habit:

When you have a ***reminder*** of what you want, create a ***routine*** of doing what you want, and have a ***reward*** for getting what you want … you have a habit! You also get what you want!

#1: My reminder is:

____

____

____

#2: My routine is:

____

____

____

#3: My reward is:

____

____

____

Let's face it, there are literally millions of things to put in your gratitude journal! When you make it a habit, you can enjoy the benefits forever.

> Show your gratitude today … right now is a good time!

I have a friend in California, who is only in his 40s, who went through some very rough times: his wife became very ill, his business failed, and life seemed unfair. He heard me speak in a public meeting about the power of gratitude. He went out and bought a gratitude journal and started his journey of wellness by expressing gratitude daily into his journal. Today, he and his wife are enjoying wellness and life! The simple daily act of expressing gratitude can truly be life changing!

Further Reading

*attractive: http://europepmc.org/abstract/MED/21191529

*others: https://scinapse.io/papers/2116855422

*lasting: https://greatergood.berkeley.edu/article/item/how_gratitude_changes_you_and_your_brain

*journal: http://happierhuman.com/benefits-of-gratitude/

Habit #9

Develop Acceptance

The reason for the habit?

– to stay focused on what you can change rather than on what you cannot

We all look for growth, improvement, and change. It's part of life, especially as we pursue wellness.

But as natural and normal as it is to expect change, what do you do when you encounter things that cannot or should not be changed? After all, not everything can be fixed, perfected, or even altered.

Self-acceptance is a very important part of well-being. When self-acceptance is lacking in someone, isn't that person also usually lacking self-worth and self-confidence? It's true! For without self-acceptance, there is little self-worth or self-confidence. They go together.

Self-acceptance is important because it enables us to accept the things we cannot change while at the same time, releasing us to focus on the changes we can make to improve our gifts, talents, skills, and the presentation of ourselves to the world.

Whether we like it or not, there are seasons or periods of time in our lives that are not going to change or respond rapidly to our efforts. We have to decide what we will accept and what we will influence with our efforts to change.

For example, if a loved one dies, there is going to be a natural period of sadness and mourning that we should accept. Life will go on, yet it will be different as well. Life has changed because that person is no longer with us, and that also needs to be accepted.

> Don't war against the past. Instead, choose to positively influence future activities and results.

Ecclesiastes 3:1-8 says it well, *"There is a time for everything, and a season for every activity under the heavens: a time to be born and a time to die, a time to plant and a time to uproot, a time to kill and a time to heal, a time to tear down and a time to build, a time to weep and a time to laugh, a time to mourn and a time to dance, a time to scatter stones and a time to gather them, a time to embrace and a time to refrain from embracing, a time to search and a time to give up, a time to keep and a time to throw away, a time to tear and a time to mend, a time to be silent and a time to speak, a time to love and a time to hate, a time for war and a time for peace"* (NIV).

Accepting Acceptance

To develop acceptance of things we cannot change is only one part of acceptance. The other part requires wisdom to recognize the times and seasons when we can try to do something about it ... but choose not to.

Now, it doesn't mean we can really change anything, it just means we choose not to spend the time, effort, and energy fighting against something we should accept. We learn from the situation while, at the same time, not allowing a victim mindset to take root in our thinking.

Accepting the things that cannot or should not be changed is actually a very important part of your wellness journey and well-being.

It is not a "quitter's mindset" at all. Let me explain.

- **Can you change the weather?** No, of course not, but you can choose what you will wear, what you will do outside, what temperature to set the thermostat inside, and more.
- **Can you change your height or bone structure?** No, not at all, but you can choose how you will eat, what you will buy at the grocery story, the level of activity you will pursue, and anything else you can do to add density to your bones.
- **Can you change the tax system?** No, but you can manage your money wisely, create savings, have insurance policies, get another job, stay out of debt, and more.
- **Can you change the fact that you will eventually die?** No, but you can choose how you will deal with death, what you will believe about eternity, how you will choose to live today, and more.

It is a matter of choosing, not a matter of changing. The challenge then is deciding what you will do throughout each day in either accepting things as they are or influencing change. What choices will you make?

In virtually every situation and experience, we face realities we cannot change while having choices we can make that are related to those unchanging realities.

I remember the moment when my wife, Susan, received a call from the medical clinic confirming the lab reports that she had breast cancer. Her cry ("Oh, no!") was chilling and the tears that followed were very traumatic. This was a difficult period of time during which she did not want to accept this medical fact.

But I also remember the moment a few days later when incredible peace came over her as she accepted the diagnosis. I heard her say, "I accept this, but I will now begin to make choices for my journey to health."

She was able to take her focus and energy away from rejecting her diagnosis and from being a victim of breast cancer and, instead, put her focus on the choices she could make. She would tell everyone, "I will do my part, the physicians will do their part, and God will do His part … and I will overcome."

There is power in knowing what to accept and what choices we can make that can lead us toward health and well-being. Today, 15 years later, Susan is going strong and has amazing health!

Here is the bottom line for all of us:

> When we accept the things we cannot change and choose instead to focus on the things that we can change, we find tremendous relief, peace, and joy.

True freedom comes from that kind of acceptance. It really does! What is more, at that point, forgiveness and gratefulness come much easier, happiness increases, and health and well-being improve.

Practice Acceptance

Have you ever stopped to make a list of things that you should accept as they are? It's actually a great exercise. Take a moment and add to this list:

Things I Cannot Change:

the weather	my height	bone structure
taxes	death	my parents
shoe size		

I realize nobody likes being forced to accept things that we feel we should have some say in. We feel demeaned, defeated, or victimized as the result.

But really, at my age, am I going to star on the football team that wins the Super Bowl? Am I going to go to become an astronaut and go to the moon? Am I going to run for president?

No, not me, but you might. In my present moment, these (and many such questions like them) are truths that I must accept.

But the key words are "present moment." Wisdom and the pursuit of life dictates that we all continue to believe in change, better days, and a bright future, but at the present moment, some things are best accepted.

Does acceptance mean that I like, want, enjoy, or support what it is I'm accepting? No it does not, but fighting against the reality that you can do nothing to stop it will do you far more harm than accepting it and moving on. (*unwanted)

Does that mean I have quit? Not at all! Nor does it mean you have quit. What it means is that you have chosen to focus on what you can change, what you can alter, and what you can achieve in your present moment. Perhaps, in the future, you will be on that Super Bowl team, on the moon, or in the White House, and that is great!

Do you see how acceptance of these things (and many others) might help bring peace, joy, and focus? It will do the same for you, so take time to make your own things-I-cannot-change list.

Consider the following in making your list:

Unchanging #1 – Accept yourself. Certain physical and personality traits are wise to accept in the present moment just as they are. After all, you can only do so much in any given day or lifetime. Can you accept that you will not always be the best, have the most, run the fastest, be the richest, or reach the highest rung on every ladder? People specialize in one area because they want to perform and be rewarded, spending incredible amounts of time and money … do you want to try to beat them? Or do you want to use your skills for something else? Accepting the reality of yourself means learning to appreciate the best of who you are while seeking to change certain thoughts and actions to avoid manifesting the worst of who you might be. With that said, we have all met someone who stated, "You are just going to have to accept me for who I am." Though that might be true for physical attributes, nobody should use that excuse for less-than-desirable behaviors. Changing certain behaviors is doable and often necessary, while physical and personality traits are best accepted so we can move on.

Unchanging #2 – Accept the reality of situations. We all must face up to what is real and choose not to live in denial or a fantasy world. Yes, some things are not as you would like them to be, but you cannot change a situation unless you first perceive the reality of it. Reality is not what you wish it to be or what you think it should be. Reality is what exists now. After you accept that, and recognize it is something that can be changed, only then can you try to actually do something about it.

Unchanging #3 – Accept nature and natural law. You cannot change the law of gravity, the killing instinct of a lion in the wild, or the course of a storm. You likely will harm yourself if you behave contrary to natural laws. Yes, there are some things you can do, such as plant a seed, tree, or crop, but you cannot predict the resulting harvest. You cannot guarantee the results. With your body, you can vaccinate, immunize, and do everything to live a life free of disease, but you cannot ensure that you will never get sick or contract a virus.

Unchanging #4 – Accept world situations. We can change a small fraction of a limited number of issues, but when things are global, political, financial, or national issues, it is much more difficult for one person to bring about changes. Nobody alive can change everything, no matter how much we want it.

Ask Yourself:

Why do I want to develop acceptance?

____

____

____

____

> **Unchanging #5 – Accept the free will of other people.** We cannot transform another person, no matter how hard we try. It is impossible to "make" another person believe, give, relate, or act in a certain way. Some people try to use force, make threats, or exert physical pressure to manipulate other people, but there is no way we can override someone else's free will.

Instead of letting ourselves be discouraged because of the things we cannot control or change, we need to accept the fact that we live in a world that is both messy and frightening … but it is limitless and exciting! You can't change that either, but in both cases, you can choose how you will focus and respond!

Each one of us should focus our energy on the choices that we alone can make, not on all the many things we cannot change. Don't fight against the wind. Set your sail, make the most of it, and enjoy the life you have been given!

Add to your things-I-cannot-change list whenever you think of something.

The point is, putting things on that list helps keep you focused on what truly matters, while letting all the other things fade away behind you.

But I Can't Let Go!

Failure to accept life's unchangeable factors causes anxiety, worry, stress, fear, and much more. Admittedly, those are not positive emotions.

Equally true is the fact we all must accept a certain degree of uncertainty in the world. If we choose not to, then we will spend unnecessary energy trying to create a false sense of security or an artificial safety zone. When we do that, our happiness evaporates, and we really have created our own emotional prison.

> To fight what you cannot change is exhausting. It sucks your energy, time, and money. Is it really worth it?
> (*decide)

Some people are weighed down by regret, but those regrets are often the result of wishing they could change something that was truly out of their control. They think, "If only..." and fill in the rest with an imagined, better reality.

But really, ask yourself:

> Do I know 100% that my imagined, much-wanted, hoped-for reality would have been better than what actually came to pass?

You cannot know, so instead of carrying around that regret for what "could have happened" but never did, let it go. Having regrets is natural, but it is completely unhealthy to live in those regrets and allow them to create stagnation or pessimism in your life.

Let it go. After all, that is the whole reason for accepting things you cannot change. Accept it so you can move on. And if you learn something in the process, all the better. (*learn)

Take the risk and let it go. You will be glad you did!

Talking personally, a tender memory of me letting go was with the passing of our dog, Pepper. She was a part of our lives for 15 years. Her passing naturally caused sadness. After several weeks of still feeling sad, our little granddaughter Autumn (just four years old) saw the pain in Meme's eyes and sang "Let It Go" in an effort to let go of the very real pain. Her little song became a reminder to let go of what we could not change. And yes, we have fond memories, but we let go of the pain, just as Autumn directed.

The Many Things You Can Change

Thankfully, life is not fixed. There are countless things that we can change each and every day. Ideally, those changes have a direct benefit on our health and wellness!

Just as we did with the things we cannot change, it is a very encouraging exercise to make a list of things you can change. I will start the list, but you can add to it with your own things that you want to do to bring about the change you desire.

Things I Can Change:

give compliments	smile	write a letter
get flowers for my spouse	try something new	spend time with a child
dress well	eat healthy	apologize
read a good book	sing in the shower	go for a walk

physical activity	give a hug	laugh
	deep breathe	

The list of things you can do is endless. The end result of your action is, of course, something you want. Consider the following:

Changeable #1 – You can change your daily habits. When it comes to the 10 habits of wellness in this book, you can make all these changes. For example, you can choose to breathe deeper, drink more pure water, get more sleep, eat more nutritiously, move more, and enjoy activity. You can make these choices regardless of what anyone around you chooses to do. Create your own habit loop with reminders, routines, and rewards to bring about the positive habits of wellness you want in your life. The end result of your choices is a better life, which you get to enjoy now and in the future!

Changeable #2 – You can choose to be happy. You are the governor of your own attitude. You are the one responsible for your own happiness.

Changeable #3 – You can choose to love yourself and others. You can choose how you will feel toward others. You can choose to encourage people, freely and generously offering help. You can choose to empathize.

Changeable #4 – You can choose to forgive yourself and others. You can choose to live free of guilt.

Changeable #5 – You can choose what you will believe. You determine your own spiritual values, and you are the creator of your own character.

Changeable #6 – You can develop your own philosophy of life. You can choose what you will learn and how you will grow personally. You can make choices to fill your life with beauty, wholeness, integrity, and goodness.

Changeable #7 – You can face and overcome your fears. What is it that you fear? Be it loneliness, failure, sickness, depression, or poverty, you can take positive steps to make friends, build relationships, enjoy better health, and create greater wealth.

Changeable #8 – You can manage at least a portion of your day. You can choose what you will do with your time and the attitudes you will have throughout your day.

Changeable #9 – You can choose to pray. Nobody can keep you from developing a relationship with your Creator.

Changeable #10 – You can choose not to complain. You can choose to trust, to walk forward in peace, to leave worrying alone, and to be free of negativity.

Your own list of things you can change is as long as you want it to be.

Make It a Habit

In every situation, you have the freedom to ask these 4 questions:

1. Is there anything I can do to improve my situation?
2. Have I done everything possible to have a positive impact?
3. Will accepting this situation and moving on help me better deal with it?

4. Did I learn from this past experience? Life learning is best done from adversity, so don't miss the opportunity!

Learn to ask yourself these questions without emotion or feelings. Keep it to "yes" or "no." Then simply do what you can do and accept the facts when you've done all you can.

> Influence others through encouragement, appreciation, and praise.

Making it a habit to measure yourself with these questions is a great practice.

Additionally, as you work to establish the habit of acceptance (and, of course, changing the things that you can), apply these 3 freedom builders to your life:

Freedom Builder #1 – Watch your language. Monitor your tone and volume and pay careful attention to what you say. Words like "should," "ought," and "must" are control words. Replace them with words and phrases such as "might consider," "perhaps," "I suggest," or "in my experience I've found." You can even ask trusted friends to help you turn "control" speech into "acceptance" speech.

Freedom Builder #2 – Thank your critics. Learn not to get angry if someone confronts, criticizes, or attacks you. Thank that person instead! Even if you address someone directly, think "thank you" in your heart. Take any good criticism and throw out the rest. Of course, there are times when criticism may not be pertinent or beneficial at all, but at least saying, "Thank you for bringing that to my attention" defuses anger and bitterness. It is also a good habit, as it then gives you time to respond in a more positive and strategic way later on, should you choose to.

Freedom Builder #3 – Speak praise and compliments. At every opportunity, even if you have to create those opportunities, freely give out genuine compliments to those around you.

Make Acceptance a Habit:

When you have a ***reminder*** of what you want, create a ***routine*** of doing what you want, and have a ***reward*** for getting what you want ... you have a habit! You also get what you want!

#1: My reminder is:

____

____

____

#2: My routine is:

____

____

____

#3: My reward is:

____

____

____

> Praise what is praiseworthy. The more you speak positive words, the more you release beneficial hormones and neurotransmitters to your body and the more it builds up other people and strengthens your relationships.

These 3 freedom builders have an uncanny way of positively and profoundly impacting your life! Put them to work for you. Ideally, if you can make them a habit, then they are yours forever.

As you work to create good habits, give yourself time to make changes. It is not always easy or quick to shift from control to acceptance. These changes may not occur overnight. Accept that reality as well!

Lastly, you now have two separate lists: 1) the things you cannot change and 2) the things you can change. Which list will you focus on? Clearly, it is the list of things you can change. The other list can be left alone.

When both of those choices become habits, you are on your way!

This daily acceptance prayer is a great reminder to developing a habit of acceptance.

> God grant me the serenity
> to accept the things I cannot change,
> courage to change the things I can,
> and wisdom to know the difference.

Further Reading

*unwanted: https://www.mindbodygreen.com/0-13730/5-things-everyone-should-know-about-acceptance.html

*decide: https://entrepreneurs.maqtoob.com/accept-what-will-not-change-change-what-you-will-not-accept-1ae7b350c142

*learn: https://www.verywellmind.com/how-accepting-emotions-can-improve-emotional-health-425368

Habit #10

Develop a Relationship with God

The reason for the habit?

– to have God's help/blessing as you pursue the wellness He wants for you

Our wellness is so physical, and yet it is also emotional, mental, and spiritual. If we focus on one area or neglect another area of our wellness, it's hard to argue that we are living as healthy as possible or living with optimal wellness.

It no longer surprises me, but I have met a lot of people over the years who are very fit, yet their bodies are constantly fighting some ailment because of issues with unforgiveness, stress, negative attitudes, or an inability to give or receive love that they have never addressed.

Every aspect of our health and well-being is important. You cannot ignore any of it because we are an integrated human being, physically, emotionally, and spiritually connected. Each part is important.

When it comes to living with optimal health and well-being, we need to be "firing on all cylinders," so to speak. We need all the parts to be working in harmony! I believe that includes our spiritual wellness.

I was extremely fortunate to have had parents and grandparents who taught me to pray and encouraged me to develop a relationship with God when I was just a child. My faith is perhaps the most important key in my pursuit of wellness because it gives meaning and purpose to all that I do, but I also feel God's love and care nurturing me on my wellness journey. I know others who feel the same.

> Virtually every aspect of spirituality and health have been researched and examined. For the studious, there are countless studies to review. (*studies)

As I was going through my health crisis, I relied heavily on God for guidance and help. I was so lost and confused because I had lived with purpose and with fitness for my entire life … but there was a raging fire of pain going through my body and desperately needed to know what to do. The doctors offered medication to lessen the pain, but they had no short-term treatments to restore my wellness.

I desperately needed help!

In the midst of my pain and anguish, I discovered that God delights in giving us forgiveness and direction. He is amazingly patient with us and delights when we want His forgiveness, help, and wisdom. He is right beside us, always a wonderfully compassionate guide to help us step-by-step as we seek His direction.

I discovered early in my life the joy of the presence of God. I always believed He was there, even in those times when I did not feel His presence. He has always been a true and loving friend who encourages, supports, and leads me through the dark times of fear and despair, as well as times of tremendous productivity and joy. I have always believed that God wants me to live a life marked by wellness and purpose.

When I committed myself to my wellness journey, I started with a simple prayer. I prayed this over and over throughout my life repeatedly, "You are His temple; I will learn to honor and respect this temple in the choices I make to nurture and nourish this temple."

Scriptures and my faith in God became a source of extra focus and increased inspiration for my restored wellness. Verses like these encouraged me every day:

- *"for I am with you, says the Lord, to save you"* (Isaiah 30:11)
- *"you shall be My people and I will be your God"* (Isaiah 30:22)
- *"the Lord appeared to me saying, Yes, I have loved you with an everlasting love, therefore with loving kindness I have drawn you, again I will build you, and you shalt be rebuilt"* (Isaiah 31:3)
- *"I will not die, but live: and declare the works of the Lord"* (Psalm 118:17)

Many of these types of scriptures became my source of hope and inspiration on my wellness journey as I searched for the essentials of wellness to nurture and nourish my body.

But, looking back, I can see countless times that God was trying to help me learn and change, but I did not recognize His guidance as I was too busy with my head down, working hard. Also, my way seemed right because of the growth and success of my efforts, so why would I want to change anything?

Unfortunately, my health had to hit rock bottom before I was really willing to listen and embrace a new way of thinking about wellness, life, and purpose. Now I know wellness is a vital force to support our God-given purpose.

Thankfully, God is patient with all of us, especially me.

9 Routines to Embrace

When it comes to a relationship with God, I have found there to be 9 simple routines to develop that help create the daily habit of furthering your relationship with God and making it vital in your wellness journey. These include:

> **Routine #1 – Communicate regularly.** Communication is the key to any good relationship, and with God, it is the very same. That is precisely what "prayer" is, just communicating with God. Admittedly, the idea of prayer intimidates a lot of people. They think they need to use a particular formula or say particular words for a prayer to be heard. In reality, God hears every person who prays to Him at any time and in any language. I want to offer a disclaimer here as this is not about

religion or about religious rituals. They are important and I encourage people to find a place of worship that is right for them, but this is for seekers of God, for in the scriptures, it says, *"Seek the lord your God and you will find Him if you will seek Him with all your heart and soul"* (Deuteronomy 4:29).

Prayer is telling God your thoughts and feelings, then listening for His response. I like to think of it as "talking things over" with God, just as I do with my wife or with friends. And did you know that God wants to be everyone's best friend?

Also, no particular tone, posture, or location is required to talk with God. He hears you, no matter where you are. He also delights in listening to us.

Routine #2 – Find a quiet place to be alone. Though God hears us no matter where we are, finding a quiet place to pray, read, or meditate is a valuable practice. Turn off the noise from sources such as cell phones, TVs, computers, and radios. Get alone, even if it's just for a few minutes.

Routine #3 – Review your emotions. If you are full of anger, frustration, anxiety, or fear, identify it. Breathe deeply, release the tension as you exhale, reject the negative emotions, and ask God for help. Receive His peace over you.

Routine #4 – Direct your heart and mind toward God. This may take a little effort with all the distracting thoughts that suddenly come to the surface as soon as we pause. Consciously set those aside. If need be, ask God to help shut them out. Pray aloud, "God, help quiet my mind and heart and put my focus on You!"

Routine #5 – Focus on God's goodness. Some people see God as a harsh judge waiting to pounce on every one of our faults and flaws, but that is not the case. God is loving, good, and kind. He is merciful, forgiving, and patient. He is dependable, true to His word, and utterly trustworthy. He is filled with joy and delights in sharing His joy with you. There are countless other positive terms to describe God, so add to this list yourself because how you perceive God affects how you see and communicate with Him.

For me, here are a few characteristics, traits, and facts about God that I believe help me desire to further my relationship with God:

Ask Yourself:

Why do I want to pray more?

____

____

____

____

- God exists, loves us, and wants to have a relationship with each one of us.
- God created us all for a divine purpose. He gave us unique gifts and talents to enable us to fulfill that purpose.
- God desires to communicate with us. He wants to hear from us and speak to us in ways we will understand.
- Each one of us was planned for God's pleasure. The moment we were born into the world, God was there as an unseen witness, smiling at our birth. He wanted us alive and our arrival gave Him great pleasure. We exist for His benefit, His glory, His purpose, and His delight! The highest purpose of our life is to bring God joy and live for His pleasure.

Interestingly, they have found that people who believe God loves them live longer after an illness diagnosis than those who believe God is looking to punish them. (*punishment)

> Spend five minutes talking to God today.

As a small yet meaningful task, I encourage you to describe God from a loving and caring point of view. Even if it stems from the perspective of how you would like God to be in your life, writing words down on paper will make a positive impact in your view of God.

Routine #6 – Be grateful. There is so much to be thankful for: life, family, friends, work, health, food, air, water, shelter, and countless other things. Grab your gratitude journal and spend a few minutes listing afresh the many things worthy of thanks. Does God not deserve credit for ultimately providing everything positive, good, and beneficial in life? While practicing the habit of gratitude, you can incorporate the habit of developing a relationship with God. That is two habits of wellness occurring in your daily life at once!

Routine #7 – Practice forgiveness. If you need to forgive someone (yourself included) or need to ask God for His forgiveness, do it without hesitation. Let go of the hurt, fears, and doubts so you can move on. You have already read about the many benefits of forgiveness. Practice the habit of forgiveness in developing your relationship with God. You will grow emotionally and spiritually and enjoy greater wellness.

Routine #8 – Tell God what you need. Ask God to resolve the problems of those you know are in need, and that includes your own needs. Remember that no need is too small or too great to discuss with God, nor is a need beyond His ability or desire to meet. Express your deepest longings to God and trust Him to answer your prayers.

Routine #9 – Discuss your purpose. God absolutely loves to see you fulfilled! I believe that with all my heart, so talk to God about your desire to accomplish your life purposes and ask Him to give you direction to pursue those things. Tell him about specific people, opportunities, needs, desires, circumstances, or situations. He cares. Talk it out, and ask for wisdom, direction, and strength to accomplish all that is in your heart.

These 9 routines in your daily life will help you develop the habit of developing a relationship with God. Using the 3 Rs habit loop (reminders, routines, and rewards) will help you better develop this wellness habit. As you can see, many different habits and routines are interconnected and help bring you rewards, such as peace, clarity, wisdom, and balance in your life. Your habits around prayer are ideally a way of life.

And your physical health? It benefits greatly from every single good habit you develop.

The Many Benefits of Prayer

There are countless benefits of prayer. I could literally write a whole book to document them. Here are a few of the benefits from prayer, as documented Biblically, scientifically, and medically:

- Reduced anxiety
- Improved relationships
- Less pain
- Decreased anger
- Lowered stress levels
- Increased efficacy of medicine and therapy
- Reduced fear
- Less worry
- Increased hope
- More peace
- Greater joy
- Improved attitude
- Elevated stamina
- Faster recovery
- Less likely to relapse
- Complete, miraculous healings

What's more, people who pray tend to take better care of themselves, exercise more, sleep better, reconcile differences and forgive more readily, and get sick less often and less severely. Some say it doesn't make sense, but this is a fact:

> People who pray feel better about themselves and others.

Prayer has also been shown to be just as effective as other meditation techniques when it comes to slowing heart rate, lowering blood pressure, and releasing healthy hormones and neurotransmitters. One study found that one group of women who received prayer were twice as likely to get pregnant than those in another group that did not receive prayer. (*pregnant)

In sum, prayer may be the most nurturing thing you can do for your total life!

Make It a Habit

Prayer is free and anyone can do it. It has the potential to be the most positive and rewarding aspect of your life. Nobody knows everything that happens when we pray, but the positive benefits we do know are abundant.

Prayer and faith in God have been validated in improving life span and quality of life. *Newsweek* published a study recently about how religious people actually live four years longer than non-religious people. (*years) And not long ago, *JAMA Internal Medicine* published an article about how religious people, by praying and having faith in God, actually increase their lifespan. (*longer)

Not only do prayer and faith in God increase our lifespan, it also improves our quality of life. Clearly, prayer does no harm, yet holds the potential to change your world forever.

How to make prayer a habit is then a natural desire. Many people have told me over the years how they combine deep breathing with prayer to make both a natural habit. This is their way of using reminders, routines, and rewards while practicing one habit to remind them of another habit.

What they do is speak a word that represents something they want to release to God as they exhale. Perhaps they want to get rid of anger, fear, or discouragement. They voice that as they breathe out. They do this for a few breaths, then pause and breathe more normally.

A few minutes later, they engage in a second round of deep breathing. This time, as they inhale, they envision breathing in the goodness of God. They focus their thoughts on God's healing power, love, mercy, forgiveness, strength, provision, and other blessings.

Make Prayer a Habit:

When you have a ***reminder*** of what you want, create a ***routine*** of doing what you want, and have a ***reward*** for getting what you want … you have a habit! You also get what you want!

#1: My reminder is:

____

____

____

#2: My routine is:

____

____

____

#3: My reward is:

____

____

____

They see themselves being filled up with the good things that God imparts to those who are in relationship with Him.

Others have told me how they write out their prayers as letters to God. It helps them focus and really pour all their emotions and feelings into the task. This gives them a greater sense of freedom and strength in return. That alone makes the habit a good one because their reward is almost instant.

> Young people with strong spirituality have more optimism, better grades, and greater persistence. They are 40% less likely to use drugs.
> (*youth)

As you grow increasingly comfortable in your relationship with God and with the habit of praying, consider asking another person to partner with you in prayer. Get together occasionally, in person or by phone, to pray for each other. I have witnessed amazing things happen to marriages, families, friendships, and yes, even people's sick bodies, when prayer becomes a component. And every part of it is good for your health and wellness!

I invite you to pray the Lord's prayer found in the Scriptures:

> "Our Father in heaven, hallowed is your name, your kingdom come, your will be done, on earth as it is in heaven. Give us day by day our daily bread, and forgive us our sins, for we also forgive everyone who is indebted to us, and do

not lead us into temptation, but deliver us from the evil one" (Luke 11:2-4 NKJ).

Further Reading

*studies: https://www.ncbi.nlm.nih.gov/pmc/articles/pmc 3671693/

*punishment: http://content.time.com/time/printout/0,8816,18 79179,00.html

*pregnant: https://www.ncbi.nlm.nih.gov/pmc/articles/pmc 2802370/

*years: https://www.newsweek.com/religious-people-live-four-years-longer-average-study-shows-976050

*longer: https://jamanetwork.com/journals/jamainternal medicine/fullarticle/2521827

*youth: http://time.com/3825083/why-kids-who-believe-in-something-are-happier-and-healthier/

Conclusion

Take the pressure off! You don't need to turn all 10 of these wellness habits into full blown habits immediately!

I suggest that you choose one wellness habit, the one that speaks to your wants and needs the most, and work to make that one habit a natural part of your life. Use the 3 Rs (reminder, routine, and reward) to help create and drive your habit.

Then, after that habit is cemented in place, choose another wellness habit to work on. Eventually, as your healthy habits increase, your body will be reaping so many benefits that you will never ever want to go back!

So take your time. And be intentional.

And step by step, you can rest assured that you are making progress toward a happier and healthier life with less illness and disease. That is the most tremendous, far-reaching reward ever!

Enjoy Your Wellness Journey

The pursuit of wellness is a lifelong quest, but it is not a destination. You cannot get there, stay, and never move again. It is a perpetual goal ... and there are countless experiences and rewards along the way. That is why it is a "journey." Since that is the case, you should make it a point to enjoy the ride!

One of the greatest ways to enjoy the 10 habits of wellness is to make them easy to do, implement, and live out. Nobody wants to do anything if it's difficult, time consuming, or complicated. I have always looked for the simple yet profound things in life. Each of these wellness habits is simple to do, yet each is equally profound! And you get to enjoy every single one of them in your life!

How to make the 10 habits of wellness as easy as possible? I suggest these 3 steps:

> **Enjoyment Step #1 – Make it easy to remember.** Whatever habit you are working on, set yourself up so you don't need to think too hard. The easier it is for you to remember, the better. For example, if you want to increase your water intake, then having a large pitcher of water sitting on the kitchen counter makes for a pretty obvious reminder. No thinking required.
>
> Or, if you are trying to boost your gratitude levels and are making it a habit to express your gratitude every time you stop at a red light on your way home from work, then a simple note stuck to your dash will make it easy. Within no time, it will be a habit!
>
> Basically, you are creating routines and reminders so that you do more of what you want.

Enjoyment Step #2 – Practice good health with someone else. You are not meant to do life alone, and that is especially true when it comes to creating the 10 habits of wellness in your life. Enlist the help of others, whether they are family or friends. It makes it more enjoyable while at the same time holding everyone accountable.

Social interaction and health go hand in hand. Being alone has adverse effects. Ever hear grandparents say that caring for their grandchildren makes them feel healthier and more active? It's true, and it works!

> Wellness is a way of thinking that becomes a way of living.

Whatever habit you want to establish in your own life, look for ways to include other people in your journey.

Enjoyment Step #3 – Know that you are worth it. Not only are you worth it, but your wellness habit will boost your positive self-image. It makes you feel good and feel good about yourself. You are worth it!

Whatever you do and whatever purpose in life you might have, you matter to others. You matter to God. You matter to yourself. Let your habits of wellness propel you to do more of what you love. You will enjoy it all the more.

> So, whether you are a parent, grandparent, caregiver, volunteer, employee, or leader in some major role, you matter to a lot of people! And your wellness is a part of your vitality and purpose. You are worth it!

The journey of wellness can start immediately, but it is a journey that lasts a lifetime. As you enjoy it along the way, there is always so much to learn, decisions to make, and options to consider.

What is more, just as health knowledge changes, so does your body change. You will need to adjust certain parts of your health routine as your body ages, as you enter into different seasons of your life, if a job change requires more or less physical activity, and so on.

> Improvement is always possible in the quest for wellness.

For example, I know a man who went from a desk job to a physically demanding job. In a few short months, he lost 30 pounds. Soon after losing all the weight, he went back to an office job. At that point, he was faced with a whole new set of choices to make for his health, how to keep the weight off, what physical activity to make part of his new routine, and more.

The wellness journey has an element of flexibility that goes with it, wherever we are and whatever we do, and that is completely normal. Just keep that in mind as you proceed.

Stay the Course

Because wellness begins in the mind, what you think about wellness results in what you actually do to enhance your wellness. As you choose to create lasting habits of wellness, I encourage you to stay the course. Your body will thank you for it!

I have found that every area of life is positively impacted by our wellness. Every physical, emotional, psychological, spiritual, and even financial area of life is affected by our level of wellness. Being vibrant and energized is sure to help! Your wellness is a vital force to support your purpose in life!

The goal for all of us is to live a happier and healthier life with less illness and disease. That is an amazing reward we get to enjoy on our wellness journey!

To learn more about wellness essentials, hear wellness experts discuss latest discoveries, and gain more benefits from the many wellness habits, visit:

www.TriVita.com/podcast

We would love to hear your story
of how your wellness habits are
helping you achieve your
personal goals and dreams.
Send your story to:

www.habitstories.com

Further Reading

Wellness Habit #1: Sleep Peacefully

*all-nighter: https://jamanetwork.com/journals/jamaneurology/fullarticle/1875833

*drowsy: https://one.nhtsa.gov/people/injury/drowsy_driving1/drowsy.html

*groggy: Van Dongen HP, Maislin G, Mullington JM, Dinges DF. The cumulative cost of additional wakefulness: dose-response effects on neurobehavioral functions and sleep physiology from chronic sleep restriction and total sleep deprivation. Sleep. 2003;26(2):117-126.

*hungry: https://www.nhlbi.nih.gov/node/4605

*depression: https://academic.oup.com/sleep/article/37/2/351/2558968

Wellness Habit #2: Breathe Deeply

*deep breathing: https://www.ncbi.nlm.nih.gov/pmc/articles/pmc5455070/)

*PTSD: https://academic.oup.com/jcem/article-abstract/98/7/2984/2537196

*live longer: Radaelli A, Raco R, Perfetti PI, et al. Effects of slow, controlled breathing on baroreceptor control of heart rate and blood pressure in healthy men. J Hypertens 2004; 22: 1361-1370.

*immune: http://options4fitness.com/options-4-relaxation/how-deep-breathing-can-help-improve-your-immune-system/

Wellness Habit #3: Drink Pure Water

*weight loss: https://www.healthline.com/nutrition/7-health-benefits-of-water#section3

*kidney: https://www.webmd.com/diet/features/6-reasons-to-drink-water

*evaporation: http://extensionpubs.unl.edu/publication/9000016361981/water/

*dry air: https://www.news.com.au/travel/travel-advice/flights/ flying-secrets-no-one-talks-about/news-story/632a8916be06c36 e39a24ea9f531e017

*water: https://www.healthline.com/health/how-much-water-should-I-drink

*food water: https://www.ncbi.nlm.nih.gov/pmc/articles/PMC 2908954/

Wellness Habit #4: Eat Nutritiously

*consistent: https://www.webmd.com/food-recipes/features/10-amazing-disease-fighting-foods

*veggies: www.ucsusa.org/11trillionreward

*obesity: https://academic.oup.com/jn/article-abstract/131/3/ 893S/4687035

*diabetes: https://academic.oup.com/jn/article-abstract/144/4/ 567S/4571642

Wellness Habit #5: Enjoy Activity

*slide: http://care.diabetesjournals.org/content/20/4/537

*choices: http://circ.ahajournals.org/content/94/4/857.full

*quality: https://www.ncbi.nlm.nih.gov/pubmed/10069785

*live longer: https://www.health.harvard.edu/promotions/ harvard-health-publications/cardio-exercise?utm_source= delivra&utm_medium=email&utm_campaign=HB20181027-Cardio&utm_id=1094082&dlv-ga-memberid=56893248 &mid=56893248&ml=1094082

Wellness Habit #6: Give and Receive Love

*married: https://www.reuters.com/article/us-health-marriage /marriage-tied-to-lower-risk-of-fatal-heart-attacks-and-strokes-idUSKBN1JE2XG

*bonus: https://www.webmd.com/sex-relationships/features/ health-benefits#1

*fighting: https://www.hyperbiotics.com/blogs/recent-articles/ how-love-improves-your-health-and-impacts-your-life *hugs: https://www.dailymail.co.uk/health/article-2266373 /Hugging-lower-blood-pressure-boost-memory.html

*lonely: http://time.com/5136409/health-benefits-love/

*destressor: https://www.huffpost.com/entry/love-health-benefits_b_3131370

*flourish: https://www.ncbi.nlm.nih.gov/pmc/articles/PMC 3537144/

*heal: https://www.ncbi.nlm.nih.gov/pubmed/15990734

Wellness Habit #7: Be Forgiving

*heart: https://www.ncbi.nlm.nih.gov/pubmed/19281923

*self-esteem: https://www.mayoclinic.org/healthy-lifestyle/adult-health/in-depth/forgiveness/art-20047692?p=1

*load: https://journals.sagepub.com/doi/abs/10.1177/194855 0614564222

*learning: https://www.hopkinsmedicine.org/health/healthy_aging/healthy_connections/forgiveness-your-health-depends-on-it

Wellness Habit #8: Practice Gratitude

*attractive: http://europepmc.org/abstract/MED/21191529

*others: https://scinapse.io/papers/2116855422

*lasting: https://greatergood.berkeley.edu/article/item/how_gratitude_changes_you_and_your_brain

*journal: http://happierhuman.com/benefits-of-gratitude/

Wellness Habit #9: Develop Acceptance

*unwanted: https://www.mindbodygreen.com/0-13730/5-things-everyone-should-know-about-acceptance.html

*decide: https://entrepreneurs.maqtoob.com/accept-what-will-not-change-change-what-you-will-not-accept-1ae7b350c142

*learn: https://www.verywellmind.com/how-accepting-emotions-can-improve-emotional-health-425368

Wellness Habit #10: Develop a Relationship with God

*studies: https://www.ncbi.nlm.nih.gov/pmc/articles/pmc 3671693/

*punishment: http://content.time.com/time/printout/0,8816,18 79179,00.html

*pregnant: https://www.ncbi.nlm.nih.gov/pmc/articles/pmc 2802370/

*years: https://www.newsweek.com/religious-people-live-four-years-longer-average-study-shows-976050

*longer: https://jamanetwork.com/journals/jamainternal medicine/fullarticle/2521827

*youth: http://time.com/3825083/why-kids-who-believe-in-something-are-happier-and-healthier/

Notes to Self

Notes to Self